The Buddha's Art of Healing

Tibetan Paintings Rediscovered

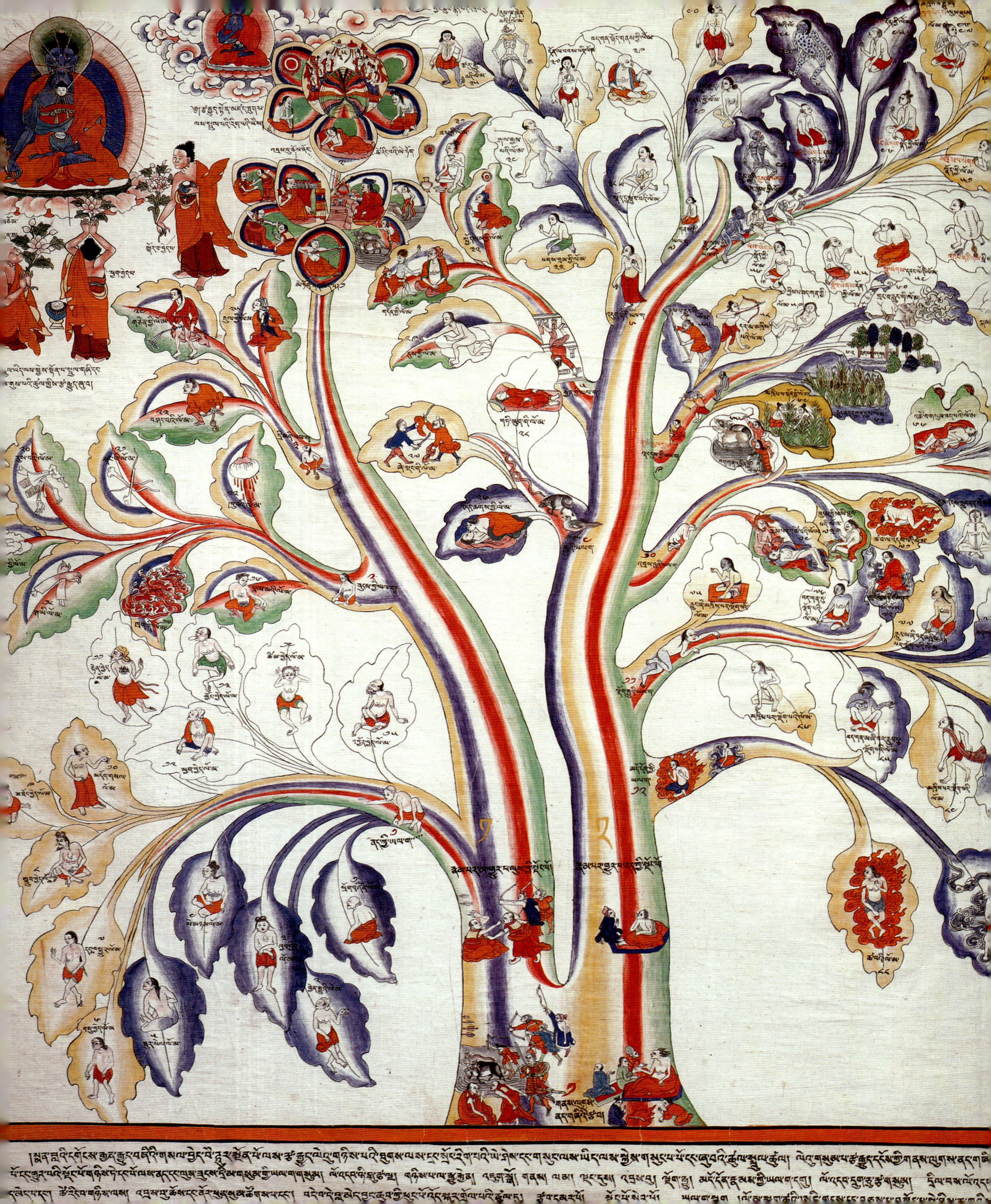

The Buddha's Art of Healing

Tibetan Paintings Rediscovered

John F. Avedon

Fernand Meyer

N. D. Bolsokhoeva

K. M. Gerasimova

Tamdin S. Bradley

Rizzoli
New York

It is the Publisher's hope that this book will encourage and invigorate the study of Tibetan medicine. The treatments and medicines outlined here are intended to be descriptive and not prescriptive, and should not be regarded as a substitute for consultation with a trained physician. Furthermore, the opinions of each author are his or her own, not necessarily shared by the other authors or by the Publisher.

First published in the United States of America in 1998 by Rizzoli International Publications, Inc.
300 Park Avenue South, New York, NY 10010

THE BUDDHA'S ART OF HEALING: *Tibetan Medical Paintings from Buryatia*
Exhibition organized by Pro-Cultura, Inc., in cooperation with the History Museum of Buryatia and the Buryat Scientific Center of the Russian Academy of Sciences.

Exhibition curated by Professor Fernand Meyer, Centre National de la Recherche Scientifique, Paris, France.

Professional services provided by the Technical Assistance Program of the American Federation of Arts.

Exhibition Venues:
Arthur M. Sackler Gallery, Smithsonian Institution, Washington, D.C.; The Aspen Art Museum, Colorado; Indiana University Art Museum, Bloomington; Michael C. Carlos Museum at Emory University, Atlanta; Museo Franz Mayer, Mexico City; The Newark Museum, New Jersey.

Frontispiece: Tibetan medical students use this Tree of Health and Disease as a schematic diagram to see, in one image, all of the eight branches of medicine (detail, pl. 2).

Library of Congress Cataloging-in-Publication Data
The Buddha's art of healing : Tibetan paintings rediscovered / John Avedon . . . [et al.].
p. cm.
"Exhibition venues: Arthur M. Sackler Gallery, Smithsonian Institution, Washington, D.C.; the Aspen Art Museum, Colorado; Indiana University Art Museum, Bloomington; Michael C. Carlos Museum at Emory University, Atlanta; Museo Franz Mayer, Mexico City; the Newark Museum, New Jersey"—
Includes bibliographical references and index.
ISBN 0-8478-2089-0 (hc). — ISBN 0-8478-2090-4 (pbk.)
1. Medicine, Tibetan—Exhibitions. I. Avedon, John F. II. Arthur M. Sackler Gallery (Smithsonian Institution) III. Title: Tibetan paintings rediscovered.
R603.T5B83 1998
610'.951'5 —dc21 97-51770
CIP

Fernand Meyer's essays translated from the French by Arthur Denner;
Bolsokhoeva and Gerasimova essay translated from the Russian by Marion Schwartz, with Catherine Fitzpatrick.

Designed by Bruce Campbell

Printed in Italy

Below: By feeling the characteristics and frequency of the patient's pulse, the doctor makes a diagnosis and establishes the best means of treatment (detail, pl. 15).

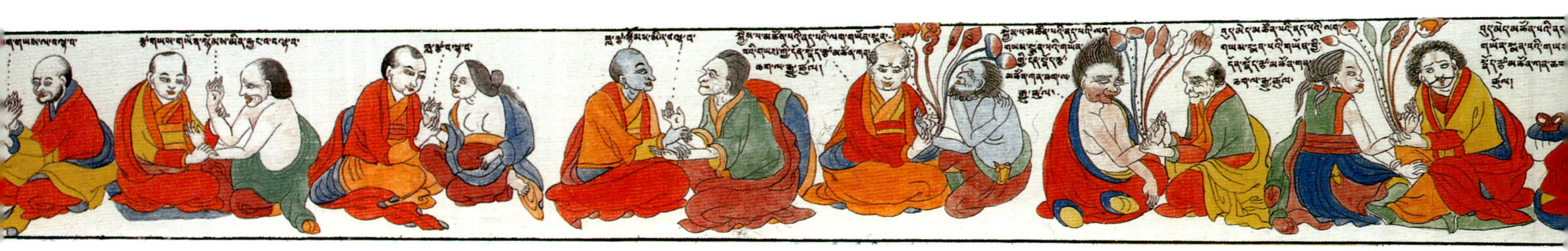

Contents

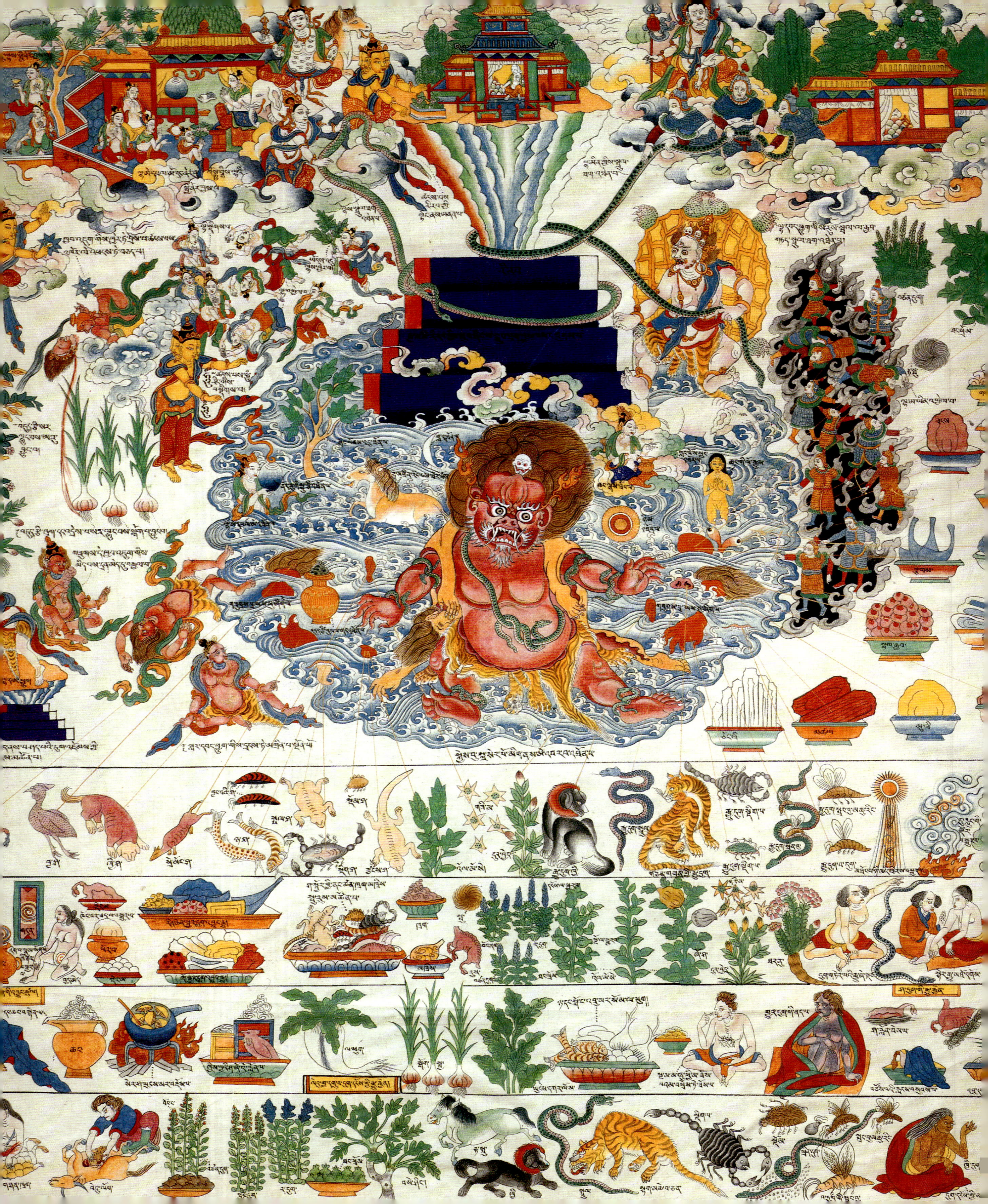

Acknowledgments

Kalakuta or Halahala, poison incarnate (detail, pl. 23).

Despite the challenge of vast distances and differences, it has been the courageous perseverance and dedication of many individuals that has given reality to *The Buddha's Art of Healing* project. The exhibition, publication, and other related events reflect a deep commitment to the ancient medical and cultural heritage of the peoples of Tibet and Buryatia.

The seed for this project was planted many years ago during a conversation with His Holiness the Dalai Lama, who encouraged us to look into the Tibetan health system. He stated on that occasion, as he has on many others, that Tibetan medicine could make a valuable and meaningful contribution to Western science and to our notions of health and healing. His Holiness's guidance and support of this project have always been invaluable. I would also like to thank Lodi Gyari Rinpoche, Tenzin Geyche Tethong, Rinchen Dharlo, Tenzin Taklha, Tenzin Choedrak, and Tsering Tashi from the Tibetan government for all their kindness, assistance, and advice.

In Buryatia, I was received with an enthusiasm, generosity, and warmth that fueled the project despite the distances. My deepest appreciation goes to Lidiya Chimitovna Nimaeva, Deputy Chairman of the Government of the Republic of Buryatia, for her support; to Gennady N. Strubinov, Minister of Culture of Buryatia; and particularly to Anatoly Piskunov, Vice-Minister of Culture, for all his help in navigating uncharted waters. We thankfully acknowledge the support we received at the Ministry of Culture in Moscow, particularly from Natalia L. Dementeva, Minister of Culture, as well as Pavel Khoroshilov and Anna Kolupaeva. Although the project was initiated under Seseg Zhambalova, former director of the History Museum of Buryatia, it was carried out under the leadership of the current director, Margarita N. Romanova. To all the museum staff my deepest gratitude. From the Buryat Scientific Center of the Russian Academy of Sciences, it was an honor to have the participation of Kseniya M. Gerasimova, Director, and especially Natalia Bolsokhoeva, our "Angel."

My very special thanks to Fernand Meyer, curator of the exhibition, who with infinite kindness and patience accommodated all my requests, and to the authors of this book, who worked on short notice and strenuous deadlines, in particular Tamdin S. Bradley, as well as Professor Gerasimova, Natalia Bolsokhoeva, and John Avedon.

The paintings were originally brought to my attention by Francesca von Thyssen von Habsburg, who opened the first doors in Buryatia, and who, under the sponsorship of the Thyssen-Bornemisa Foundation, was able to bring Robert Bruce-Gardner from the Courtauld Institute to Ulan-Ude to conduct conservation of the paintings. I particularly wish to thank the earlier supporters of the project: Lama Tenzin Samaev, Bernard Druger, Richard Gere, Jodie Eastman, Bokhara Legendre, and Carol Corcoran, as well as others who lent their wise counsel and encouraging support: Mary and Richard Lanier, Nina Reznick, Kathleen Connors, Gregory Kruglack, Philip Webber, Carol Savvas, Mary Daly, Herbert Schwabl, Michael Afanasiev, Garech Browne, Yanki Tsering, Alberta Brambatti and Joe Pantigoso. I would also like to specially thank Irina Pantaeva and Roland Levin for their continued help and resourcefulness. My gratitude goes also to Elena Orpokova, Pro-Cultura's coordinator in Moscow, without whom the most complicated logistics of the project in Russia could never have been carried out.

Special thanks to the doctors and scholars on the Advisory Committee, who so generously gave of their time and advice, especially John F. Avedon, Michael J. Balick, Herbert Benson, Dan Goleman, Jeffrey Hopkins, Fredi Kronenberg, Robert Livingston, Woodson C. Merrel, Dean Ornish, Andrew Weil, and Kenneth G. Zysk.

Perhaps most is owed to Michael Wilkinson, who was always there to help pick up the pieces and encourage us to keep trying, without whose advice and financial support this project could not have been carried out and to whom this book is dedicated.

This project was made possible through the generosity of Michael Wilkinson, the Gere Foundation, the Tara Foundation, Bernard Kruger, John and Jodie Eastman, Judith McBean Cosper, Duferco Ltd., Padma Ltd., the Trust for Mutual Understanding, the Fetzer Institute, and CSC, Inc.

Finally, my deepest gratitude to Martha Kaplan and to Barbara Einzig and Liana Fredley, who accomplished a monumental task, as well as to Sarah Fogel and Diane Rosenblum at the American Federation of Arts for all their help.

Lastly, my final words of thanks are for Nonie King, whose help, support, and advice have always been invaluable.

Anna Souza
Director, Pro-Cultura, Inc.

Museum Statement

The Matvei Nikolaevich Khangalov History Museum of Buryatia was founded in 1923 in Ulan-Ude, the capital of Buryatia. In 1958 it was named in honor of Khangalov (1858–1918), a prominent Buryat ethnographer whose work was dedicated to the preservation of the spiritual values and artistic culture of his people. Today the museum's collections number more than two hundred thousand objects, including a valuable collection of Buddhist scroll paintings, sculptures, masks, costumes, and musical instruments. Some of the rarest of these artifacts are the Buddhist canonical books of *Kangyur* and *Tangyur*, and the *Atlas of Tibetan Medicine,* which the museum staff saved from destruction during Stalin's campaign against religion in the thirties. The museum is proud of the fact that despite the difficulties inherent in our situation we have carefully and lovingly preserved the paintings of the *Atlas* as part of the rich legacy of Buddhism in Russia.

Buddhist lore tells of certain teachings of the Buddha that are hidden away in underwater palaces, guarded closely by water deities until humankind is ready to receive them. Though the *Atlas* was originally intended to be used and studied widely as an instructional guide to the Tibetan medical system, for many reasons the scrolls have never before been exhibited to the public. Perhaps it can be said that these paintings are like the mythic teachings of the Buddha, and only now are we all capable of understanding and appreciating the art of healing they represent.

This international exhibition, made possible by the untiring efforts and sacrifices of courageous, forward-looking people throughout the years, will at last bring this rare cultural artifact into the light. We wish to express our utmost gratitude to Pro-Cultura, Inc., especially its director, Anna Souza, and to all the museums participating in this historic exhibition.

The *Atlas* is not only an extraordinary work of art but also holds the keys to the practical application of Tibetan medicine. It is our hope that this exhibition and publication will help foster the development of cultural ties worldwide, contribute to a greater understanding of the ancient artistic and medical traditions of central Asia, and serve the cause of strengthening peace and friendship among peoples.

MARGARITA N. ROMANOVA
Director, The History Museum of Buryatia

Message from the Republic of Buryatia

The vast expanse of the Siberian region may seem to have been asleep throughout the centuries, but its history has been far from quiet. Siberia occupies seventy-five percent of the Russian territory, with almost thirty-five million people inhabiting the area. The Buryat Republic, between Lake Baikal and Mongolia in southern Siberia, has a population of about a million people of more than one hundred different nationalities—Russian, Buryat, Evenk, Tatar, German, Ukranian, and others. Buryatia has one of the most beautiful and dramatic landscapes on earth. Here winters are long and cold, summers are hot and dry, and the sky is eternally blue. This ancient country has a rich history; great movements of people have passed through it. Buryatia is the gateway between the Gobi desert and the Tibetan range, the Mongolian steppes and the snow-capped peaks of the Himalayas. Early tribes of hunters were replaced by Huns, who were succeeded by warriors of the powerful Syanbi tribes, who themselves experienced the destructive forces of Genghis Khan in the thirteenth century.

Buddhism was brought to Buryatia by monks from Tibet. It is known that in 1712 about 150 lamas came from Mongolia to Buryatia, and in 1741 Buddhism was officially recognized by the Russian Government when the Empress Elizaveta Petrovna legalized the existence of 11 datsans, the Buddhist monasteries. The empress herself was considered to be an incarnation of the great Buddhist deity Tara.

Datsans became great centers of education and culture. They developed a distinctive medical tradition, book-printing, philosophy, astronomy, astrology, arts, and other sciences. Agvan Dorzhiev, the spiritual teacher of the Thirteenth Dalai Lama around the turn of the century, and Piotr Badmayev, the personal physician of the last Russian czar, were educated in these datsans.

The unique *Atlas of Tibetan Medicine* displayed in this exhibition is housed at the History Museum of Buryatia in Ulan-Ude, the capital of Buryatia. Buryat scientists studying the remedies presented in these paintings and in early Tibetan medical texts have discovered medicines that are remarkably successful, particularly in treating chronic diseases. Tibetan medicine is alive and well and continues to play an important role in Buryatia today.

It gives us great pleasure that through this exhibition the world now has an opportunity to get acquainted with the traditions, culture, and history of Buryatia. The people of our republic are warm and hospitable, and we cordially invite you to visit our ancient homeland.

Lidiya Chimitovna Nimaeva
Deputy Chairman of the Government of the Republic of Buryatia

Foreword by His Holiness the Dalai Lama

Along with Tibetan Buddhism, Tibet's most important and enduring legacy is its unique and highly skilled medical tradition. Practiced successfully for more than a thousand years, and for centuries sought after by many of Tibet's neighboring countries in Asia, the system has proven effective in so many areas that this is the one aspect of Tibetan culture that even the Chinese have actively preserved and promoted. So successful is Tibetan medicine that where it is practiced—particularly in China, Nepal, Sikkim, Bhutan, northern India, Mongolia, and other areas of Buddhist Russia—Tibet has come to be known as the Land of Medicine.

I believe that the Tibetan medical system can contribute substantially to maintaining a healthy mind and a healthy body. Like the traditional Indian and Chinese systems, Tibetan medicine views health as a balance that can be disturbed by circumstances such as diet, lifestyle, and seasonal and mental conditions, giving rise to different kinds of disorders. A Tibetan physician employs his own senses to examine the individual's general balance of health as a whole. Treatment involves dietary and behavioral advice and medication. Medicines, which have few side-effects, are obtained from natural sources such as herbs, minerals, and organic products, and are prepared under controlled conditions.

As an integrated system of health care, Tibetan medicine can offer allopathic medicine a different perspective on health. However, like other scientific systems, it must be understood on its own terms, as well as in the context of objective investigation. The benefits of further exchanges between Tibetan and Western doctors, scientists, and scholars are substantial, and in practice Tibetan medicine can offer Westerners another approach to achieving happiness through health and balance.

The Buddha's Art of Healing project, with its exhibition, catalogue, and the first international congress on Tibetan medicine, will certainly create a greater awareness of our medical tradition. In particular, it gives me pleasure that the public will be able to see for the first time the unique set of medical paintings that were taken from Tibet to Buryatia for the purpose of training doctors in the Tibetan tradition. This project will make clear the importance of preserving and studying Tibet's ancient medical tradition, not just for the sake of the Tibetan people, but for all humanity.

May 16, 1997

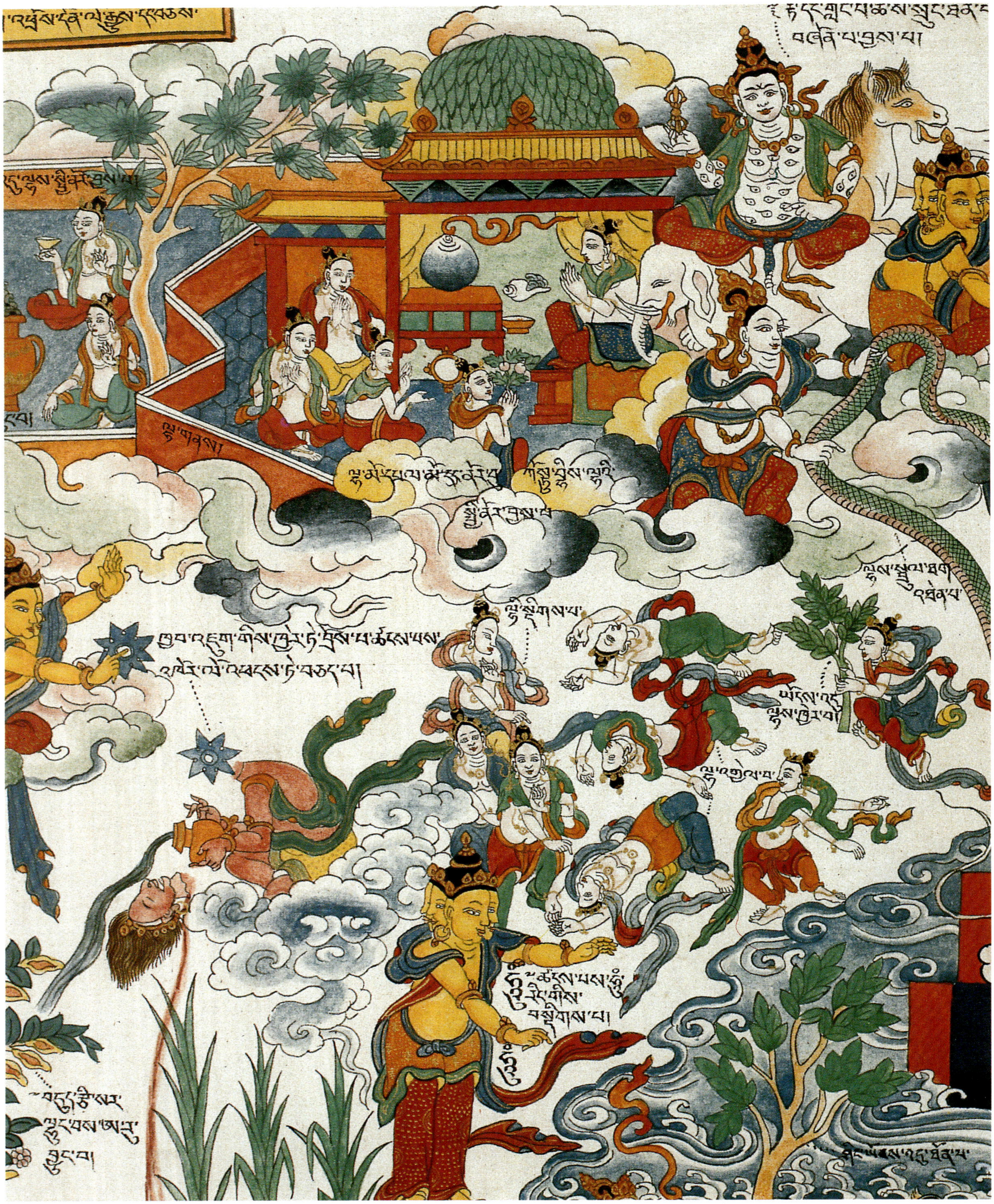

Introduction

The realm of the gods, who, unlike the anti-gods, are capable of drinking wine. Here they enjoy themselves beneath the tree of wish-fulfillment (detail, pl. 23).

The *Buddha's Art of Healing* presents forty paintings from the world's most important collection of Tibetan medical art: seventy-seven thangkas illustrating a seventeenth-century medical text called the *Blue Beryl*—an encyclopedic commentary on *sowa rigpa,* Tibet's ancient "science of healing." These paintings comprise a magnificent bridge to a heretofore hidden body of knowledge: a medical system whose unique theory and practice, developed in isolation for almost two thousand years, is just now being introduced to the West.

Tibetan medicine began in the great Buddhist monasteries of northern India. Introduced to Tibet in the first century B.C.E., it developed over eight hundred years until the first national medical college, called Melung, Country of Medicine, was founded in the eighth century by King Trisong Detsen. Nine hundred years later Sangye Gyamtso, the Regent of the Fifth Dalai Lama, systematized medical practice in a second national college, Chagpori, Iron Hill, in Lhasa. To provide medical treatment throughout Tibet and Mongolia, the Thirteenth Dalai Lama founded Tibet's third central medical college, Mendzekhang, Medicine House, in 1916. Mendzekhang was the model for numerous regional medicial schools, such as the college—at Atsagat in the Transbaikal area of Russia—that once housed the paintings in this volume. Hence, the education offered in Mendzekhang, prior to its destruction by communist China in 1959, best illuminates the rich heritage of Tibetan medicine.

Mendzekhang occupied a large building in western Lhasa. Medicinal plants grew before its main gate; herbs dried, waiting manufacture into drugs, along its courtyard, corridors, and rooftops. Amidst their pungent aroma, some three hundred students—drawn from monasteries, district headquarters, and military camps—pursued an eleven-year training in memorization, academic study, and internship.

The day began at four in the morning to the rapid, sing-song trilling of younger students memorizing the 1,140 pages of the four medical tantras: the root texts, supplemented by hundreds of commentaries, pharmacology catalogues, and illustrated texts that codify Tibetan medicine. After quizzes, congregational prayers, and breakfast, college members joined doctors from Chagpori on rounds in the city while long lines of patients were treated, free of charge, at Mendzekhang itself. Classes ran from noon until an early dinner, after which a five-hour debate session—the crucible for refining knowledge throughout Tibet's higher academic institutions—animated the central courtyard until ten o'clock.

Having memorized the tantras, the thirteen-year-old students began classes. Their curriculum was illustrated by a diagram called the Tree of Health and Disease (see plates 2, 13, and 19), a schematic tree—learned from being assembled with sticks, colored thread, and bright plastic buttons—of 3 roots, 9 trunks, 42 branches, 224 leaves, 3 fruits, and 2 flowers. When all 156 chapters of the *Four Tantras* were collated to corresponding parts of the tree, eleven subjects—progressing from anatomy and physiology through advanced courses in pathology, treatment, and diagnosis—were pursued over four years. The first class introduced the central theory of bodily humors.

Tibetan medicine ascribes all metabolic function to three physical humors: wind *(rlung)*, bile *(mkhris-pa)*, and phlegm *(bad-kan)*. Wind—controlling movement, circulation, respiration, and cognition—is described as "rough, hard, cold, subtle, and motile"; bile—regulating digestion, sight, and skin tone—is "light, oily, acrid, and hot"; phlegm—promoting, among other properties, cohesiveness—is "sticky, cool, heavy, and gentle." Respectively dominating old age, adulthood, and youth, wind moves through the skeleton, bile through the blood, and phlegm in the flesh, fat, and generative fluids. Disease results when one or more of the different types of each humor becomes imbalanced.

Humoral theory is most extensively applied in pathology. Instructors taught the causes, symptoms, and complications of some 1,616 divisions of a potential 84,000 diseases in terms of single, double, and triple humoral imbalance, an approach that included pathogens but emphasized the body's own variable response to disease. Only when the full range of human illness was fathomed—and applied to subdisciplines such as embryology, pediatrics, women's medicine, and signs of impending death—did students proceed to the equally prodigious subject of treatment.

Tibetan medicine fights illness with emetics, purgatives, moxibustion, cauterization, bloodletting, and acupuncture, which is believed to have originated in Tibet, whence it spread to China via Mongolia. (Major surgery has been prohibited since the eighth-century death, during a heart operation, of King Muni Tsenpo's mother.) However, the system's primary means of treatment is herbal. Following formulas conceived by generations of physicians, Mendzekhang's pharmacy compounded plants, animal products, and minerals into more than a thousand standard medicines. The college's future doctors were required to have a thorough knowledge of Tibet's unique flora.

At the start of each July, classes traveled to Dhakyaba, a nearby region of alpine meadows considered ideal for gathering herbs. Pairs of students, followed by a groom and pack animal, spent seven weeks—shifting location every three days—collecting plants. Thirty types of plants were harvested; medicinal substances in the roots, stems, flowers, leaves, and fruit of hundreds of less important herbs were also sought. Halfway through the summer, large wooden crates containing rare plants packed in ice and snow arrived at Mendzekhang from outlying districts. Many of these were used to fabricate the most powerful medicines in the Tibetan pharmacopoeia, called, for their pervasive effects, Precious Pills. The weakest of the seven Precious Pills contains eighteen compounds; the strongest, known as the King of Medicines, is produced over three months of continual labor from 165 different ingredients.

The most difficult subject in a doctor's training was diagnosis. Unlike academic study, the three trunks, eight branches, and thirty-eight leaves of the diagnostic root (see plate 13) could only be learned from lengthy practice. Though nine aspects of a patient's urine were analyzed, physicians probed illness through pulse diagnosis, an immensely sophisticated assay explained in thirteen sections of the Subsequent Tantra, the last of the four medical tantras.

Pulse diagnosis took a year to study and a decade to master. Ideally performed at dawn—when hot and cold forces are best balanced—the diagnosis monitors both overall physiology and the condition of individual organs through dozens of subtle fluctuations in blood flow. When performed too close to vital organs, pulse diagnosis is said to resemble "talking to someone by a waterfall"; if attempted too far away, it proves no better than "receiving messages from distant merchants." Accordingly, Tibetan doctors listen to the pulse—like "a voice shouting across an open field in summer"—on the radial artery at the wrist. The Subsequent Tantra says that "just as an astute businessman can discern the origin and make of wares at a marketplace, so the pulse, if read at the radial artery, can exhibit the condition of the hollow and full organs."

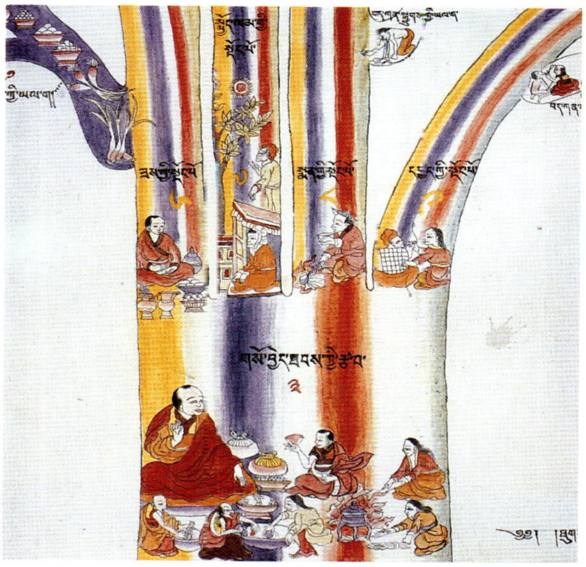

The root of treatment has four trunks: diet, conduct, medicine, and external therapies (detail, pl. 19).

Required to keep their fingertips "smooth, sensitive, without scars, and pliable," physicians press the index, middle, and ring fingers of one hand to the skin, flesh, and bone of the patient's wrist, then switch hands to examine the other arm. They first register the "constitutional" and "seasonal" pulses, traits that display the individual's dominant humor and the climate's influence. Pulse rate is measured to determine overall health, after which the duration and severity of illness is determined through one of six hot and cold pulse qualities: "strong, ample, rolling, swift, tight, and hard" or "weak, deep, declining, slow, loose, and hollow." Thereupon, the humors are read and specific conditions isolated. If worms are present, for example, the pulse feels "flat" and seems to "knot" as it beats; if bacteria, the pulse shows an "incomplete" aspect, with "sudden, irregular, and unpredictable cessation in rhythm." Leprosy produces a pulse that "quivers" and "contracts" like "a person who limps"; wounds cause a "bulky, hard, and quick" pulse; pregnancy creates a pulse that can reveal the fetus's sex when read after the sixth week. Finally, twelve major organs are checked through the outer and inner sides of the doctor's six monitoring fingertips; for example, the physician uses his right index finger to check the heart and small intestine, while his middle finger surveys the spleen and stomach. At Mendzekhang, students were expected to report the age, nature, and severity of any humoral imbalance, which organs were most affected, and in what manner, within the course of one hundred breaths.

Pulse diagnosis is also used to reveal future health. A patient is deemed terminal if either the "changing" or "irregular" death pulses appear: the former "flutters like a flag in the wind," the latter resembles "a vulture who, attacking a bird, stops, plunges, quickly beats its wings, stops again, and resumes flight." Death from a combined wind/bile disorder is heralded by a pulse like "a fish leaping from the water to catch a fly and quickly shimmering back." A fatal phlegm/wind disease pulses like "the pecking of a hen eating grain"; a deadly triple humoral imbalance approximates "the saliva of a drooling cow moving in the wind." Three days of life remain if the liver or gall bladder pulse is missing; two, if the large intestine and lung pulses are absent. Physicians are believed to have perfected their craft when they are able to predict the lifespan of a healthy person, identify various types of spirit possession, and use the seven "amazing pulses" to foretell the course of an illness.

On completing studies, Mendzekhang's students undertook a four-year internship, a period of intensive practice that soon revealed both the efficacy and limits of their science. The interns found that chronic and multiple disorders were especially responsive to a restoration of humoral balance. In addition, a number of major disorders could be successfully combated, including coronary disease, arthritis, hepatitis, Parkinson's disease, diabetes, ulcers, the common cold, senility, infertility, and fifty-four types of cancer—one of eighteen new diseases predicted by

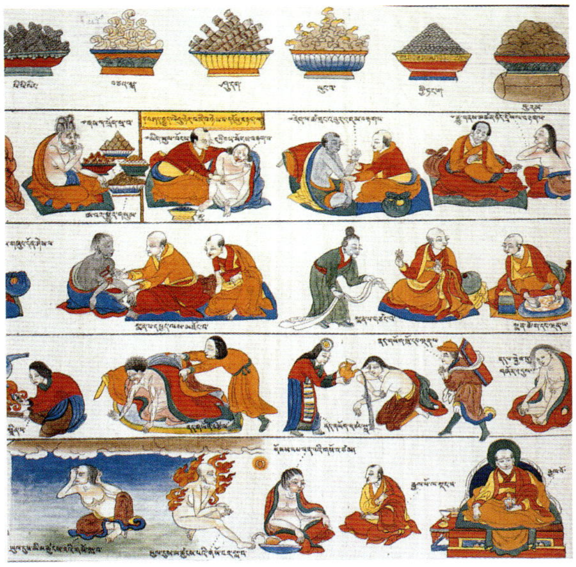

This detail (pl. 20) illustrates how a good physician, good medicine, caring nursing, and an attentive patient can be all that is required for cure.

the Buddha to arise from environmental pollution and unethical conduct. Though Buddhist morals discouraged their prescription, doctors possessed two types of birth control: one effective for a year, the other for life. A more arcane branch of medicine, called *chu-len* ("extracting the essence"), combined meditation with the drawing of nourishment from seeds and flowers to foster rejuvenation and longevity. Epilepsy and paralysis, the young doctors soon discovered, were their most recalcitrant foes.

Mendzekhang concluded its academic year with publicly held final exams. Hundreds of family members, friends, and local villagers joined the college in Dhakyaba, where a large tent was erected to conduct the test. Inside, Mendzekhang's principal—a renowned doctor named Khyenrab Norbu (1883–1962) who was the personal physician of the Thirteenth Dalai Lama—officiated from a high throne as professors led groups of three students past two hundred plants displayed on stacks of cotton-covered wood. When each examinee had attempted to identify the class, species, and active parts of every plant, the group was guided out the back of the tent, their scores tabulated, and the remaining candidates informed of the results—a practice which greatly heightened tension, as prospective graduates typically failed up to five times before correctly describing a majority of the specimens. Following the exam, students were shown their mistakes, ranked, and released for a picnic. The first- and second-place winners received long silk scarves embroidered with the motto "Luck in the day and night." Less successful competitors garnered more dubious honors. The fifth from last was given a blue medicine bag and proclaimed "Carrier of the Medicines"—a barb equivalent to nurse; the fourth, called "The Doorman," was made to guard the tent's entrance in the black robes of a government servant; the third, costumed as a muleteer, drove the two worst candidates—dubbed the White and Black Donkeys—bellowing and braying under halters, reins, bells, and loads of plants around the much-amused crowd. The next day the college returned to Lhasa for an elaborate offering ceremony in the Central Cathedral and then broke for a week's vacation.

Both Mendzekhang and Chagpori—together with virtually every other Tibetan institution—were destroyed by China's 1959 invasion and subsequent military suppression of Tibet. When a hundred thousand Tibetans followed the Fourteenth Dalai Lama into exile in 1959, only three Mendzekhang-trained doctors were among them.

In 1961, the Dalai Lama instructed Yeshi Dhonden, a leading physician of Mendzekhang's 1949 class, to found the Tibetan Medical Institute (TMI) in Dharamsala, India, the capital of the Tibetan diaspora. Dr. Dhonden began the institute with a twenty-bed hospital and fifteen students to whom he taught a condensed seven-year curriculum. During the past thirty-six years, TMI has greatly enlarged its hospital, college, and pharmacy, built thirty-six branch centers and graduated 167 doctors who annually care for more than half a million patients. In 1992 Trogawa Rinpoche, a Chagpori-trained physician, founded the Chagpori Medical Insitute in Darjeeling, India. Tibetan medicine has also been revived in Tibet. In the 1970s, China permitted surviving Tibetan physicians to open the Hospital of Tibetan Medicine in Lhasa. Its 127-member staff treats almost a thousand patients a day, and its medicines, grown on high-altitude farms, are sold under Chinese labels throughout the People's Republic.

Dr. Dhonden introduced Tibetan medicine to the West during a 1974 tour of the United States. Since then, Tibetan physicians have visited teaching hospitals, provided drugs for laboratory research, and sought to stimulate dialogue with their Western peers. While significant exchange is only now beginning, interest in Tibetan medicine has rapidly grown.

"I went to observe Dr. Dhonden with some healthy skepticism," remarked Richard Selzer, a Yale surgeon who attended an early demonstration of pulse diagnosis. "I was surprised and elated by what I found. It was as if he were a human electrocardiogram machine interpreting the component parts of the pulse. We have nothing like it in the West. It's a dimension of medicine we have not yet realized."

"Over one third of our pharmacopoeia comes from plants and microorganisms," observed Gerald Goldstein, an oncologist who hosted Dr. Dhonden at the University of Virginia. "These are just the sort of materials Tibetans have acquired extensive experience with. Some of their medicines are definitely going to be active."

"Tibetan formulas have proven efficacious in controlled, double-blind studies," stated Herbert Schwabl, an Austrian biophysicist who heads a Swiss firm that manufactures Tibetan medicines. "They clearly initiate healing by providing what the diseased body lacks, by making it 'whole' once more. If we could translate Tibetan principles into Western techniques, many new methods of treatment would undoubtedly result."

"Tibetan and Western medicine begin from completely opposite standpoints," said Dr. Dhonden, comparing traditions. "Western scientists look through a microscope to discover the disease-causing agent; Tibetan physicians first consider the patient's disposition in terms of wind, bile, and phlegm. The difference makes for strengths and weaknesses in each. While we lack many quick-acting symptomatic treatments, modern medicine's ignorance of humoral function prevents it from establishing a clear view of the causes and conditions governing disease. Each of us," Dr. Dhonden judiciously concluded, "has something of value to learn from the other."

Only three sets of the *Blue Beryl* paintings are known to still exist. While Chagpori's copy was most likely destroyed in the 1959 artillery barrage that leveled its hilltop campus, Mendzekhang's and the Dalai Lama's—kept in the Norbulingka or summer palace—survived. As explained in the ensuing essay by Bolsckhoeva and Gerasimova, Atsagat's paintings barely escaped the Stalinist purges of the 1930s. Like the *Blue Beryl* paintings, Tibet's vast treasury of medical knowledge almost perished—but did not. *The Buddha's Art of Healing* beautifully preserves and will undoubtedly promote Tibetan medicine's unique potential to benefit humanity.

JOHN F. AVEDON

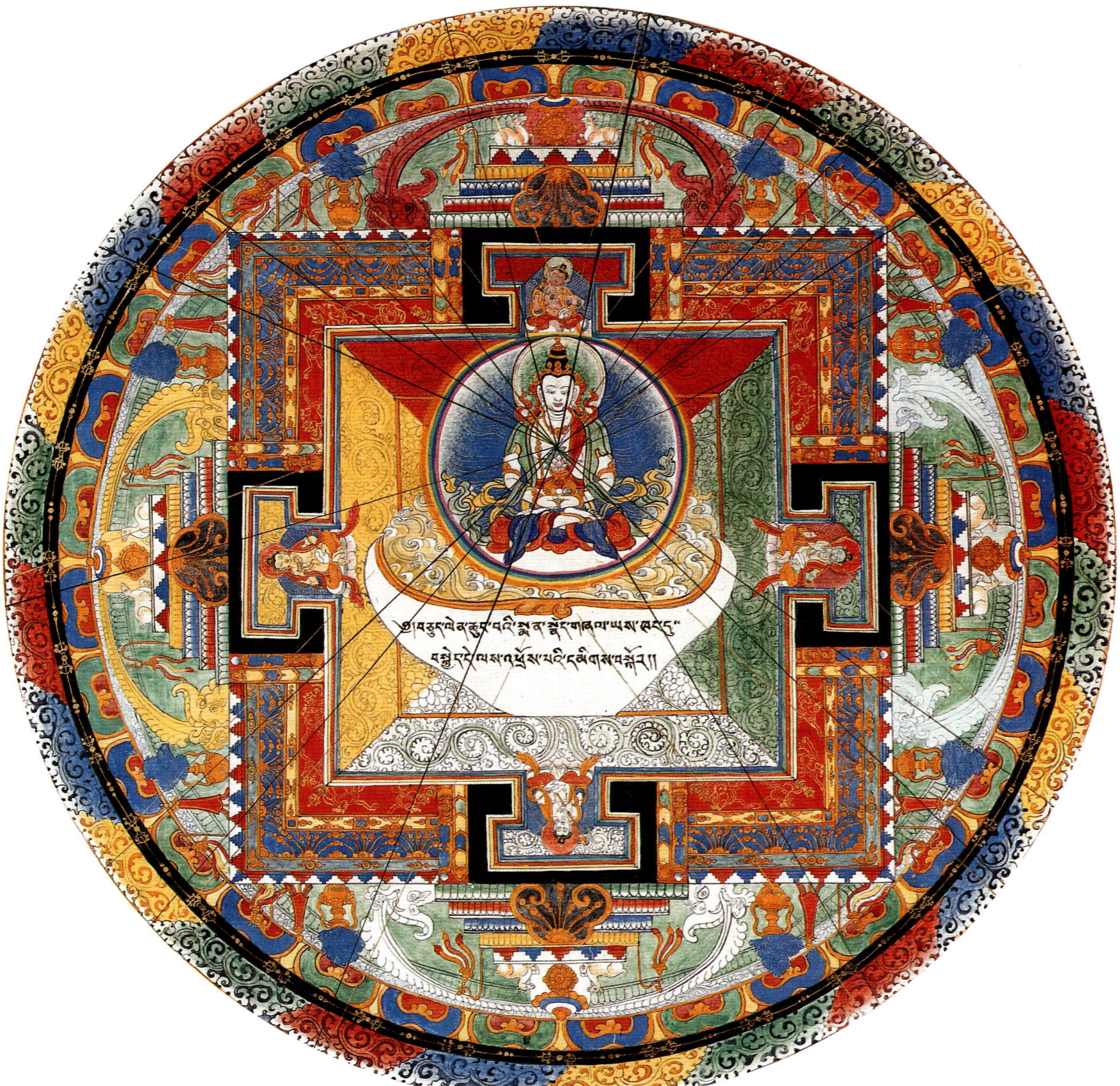

The Buddha's Art of Healing

TIBETAN PAINTINGS REDISCOVERED

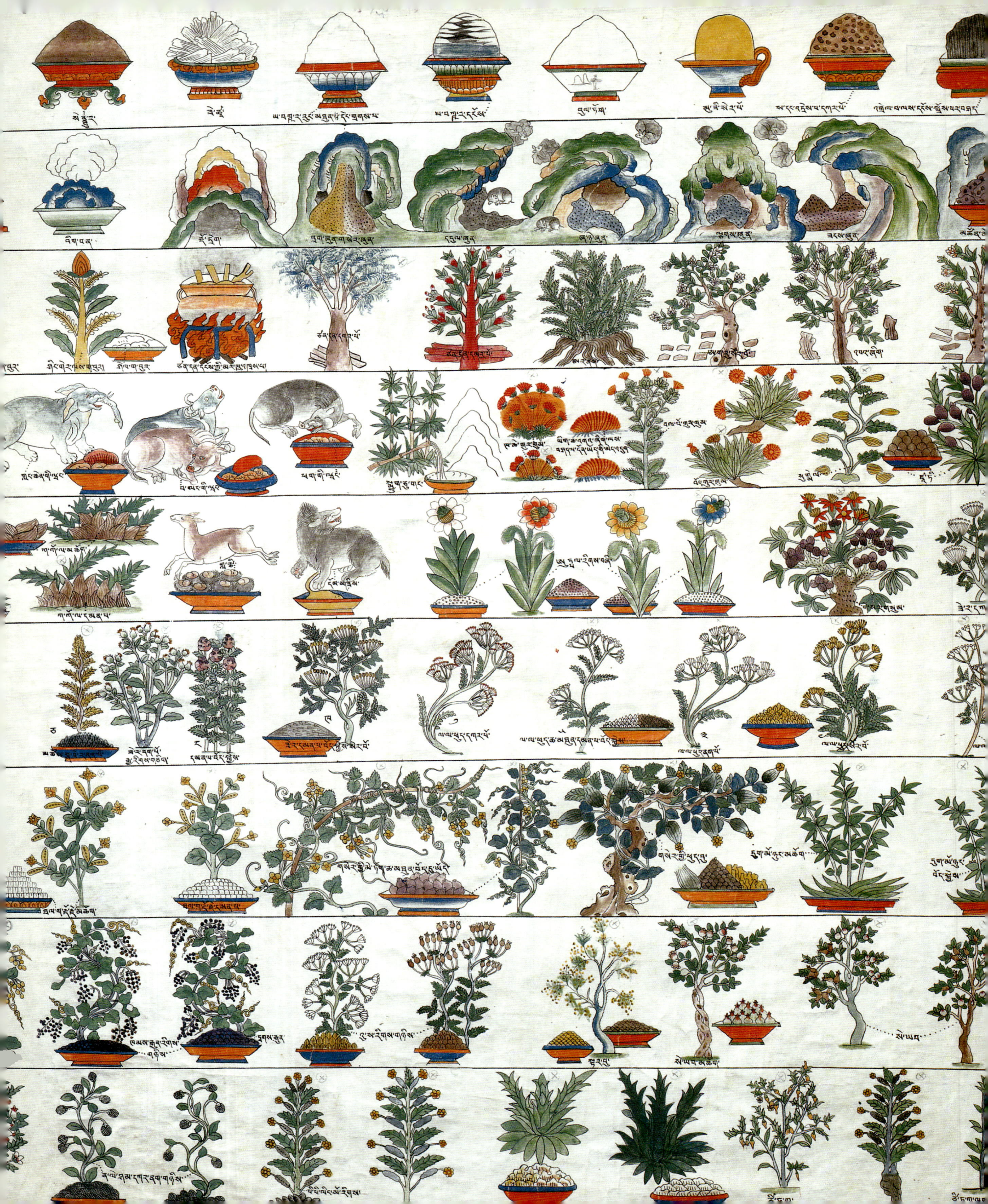

The History and Foundations of Tibetan Medicine

On this great occasion of the great teachings of the Master, each group understood in its own unique way.
— *The Four Tantras*

Ancient Medicine in Historical Perspective

Illness is a misfortune that has afflicted humanity since our beginnings. In human experience, it belongs with the larger categories of evil, calamity, and disorder that like disease threaten the integrity of both the individual and the group to which he belongs. Like birth and death, illness is that sort of event, at once individual and social, imposed by the biological condition of man. However, illness differs in that one generally spontaneously recovers—which tends to be credited to the therapeutic enterprise; illness recurs within one's lifetime.

Tibetan medicine's primary means of treatment is herbal, using many medicinal substances found in the roots, stems, flowers, leaves, and fruits of hundreds of plants (detail, pl. 25).

Since the dawn of time, people have tried to interpret and deal with illness just as they have coped with other individual or collective hard times such as natural disasters, unsuccessful hunting expeditions, crop failures, childlessness, and death before one's time. Yet because illness takes place at the most profound level of the suffering body, it calls into play very strong emotions and triggers social processes that can assume complex dimensions. Furthermore, because the disease-event is pernicious, unexpected, and apparently selective, it drives the afflicted and those around them to seek out, sometimes with the aid of specialists, not only an effective course of action against the disease but also an explanation that can give meaning to the event. Such an explanation works not only through its correlation with a degree of truth—its scientific or even empirical verifiability—but also through how well it harmonizes with the subjective experience of the patient and his own ideas of his relationship with others and with the visible and invisible worlds. In this search for meaning, man first turned to explanatory models that attributed illness to beings—gods, demons, spirits, ancestors, sorcerors—with evil intentions toward their victims; such explanations seemed to make sense of the singularity of each individual case. This kind of reason for illness could be best found out through such methods as divination or trance rather than through observation of symptoms. Thus throughout a long period of human history, the task of treating illness fell to laymen or specialists—soothsayers, shamans, and priests—whose therapeutic arsenal consisted of the same sorts of intervention as were applied against all other forms of misfortune.

In time, there gradually emerged a kind of specialist whose knowledge and practices centered on a particular category of affliction that strikes the body: disease, that which is biological misfortune. With this new type of healer, the explanatory model became more oriented toward naturalistic causes such as climate, diet, lifestyle, and emotional disposition, impersonal factors attributed to no one; their meaning and impact are of a universal rather than a personal nature. Attention also shifted to the pathogenic processes themselves: humoral imbalances, blockages

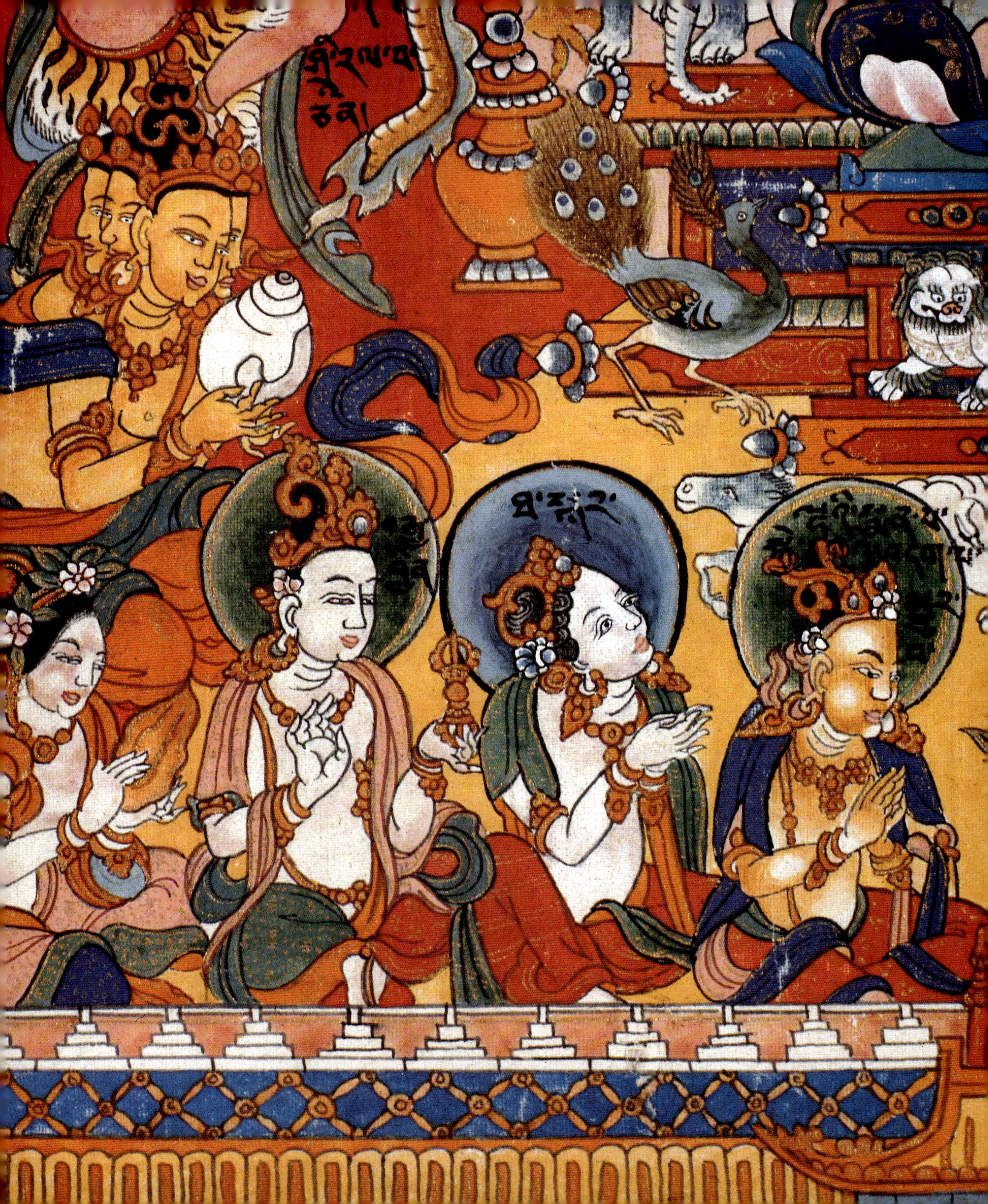

or deviations of bodily flows, corruption of the bodily fluids. This new orientation, which gave birth to the ancient learned medical traditions and their vast bodies of literature, constituted an important break with the more archaic tendency described above, with its magico-religious interpretations of disease. This earlier tendency did not disappear, however, but persisted alongside more strictly medical theories and practices. Nonmedical specialists thus continued a parallel tradition that offered alternatives responding to needs that medicine alone often could not meet. At the same time, medical practitioners themselves continued to incorporate into their medical writings and into their practice ideas and techniques that belonged to the realm of magic and religion.

Prajapatidaksa, physician of the gods, a member of the original audience when the Healing Buddha first explained the medical teachings. Lord of Living Beings, he is among the founders of the art of therapy (detail, pl. 1).

The first medical traditions to produce a written body of literature developed gradually around the Mediterranean, in India, and in China in the centuries preceding the birth of Christ. These medical systems, whose grounding in a written corpus qualifies them as learned traditions, share four fundamental features, despite their distinct origins.

1. All of them ascribe their origins to texts attributed to historical or legendary figures who came to acquire a heroic stature as emblematic founders of these traditions: Hippocrates in the Greco-Roman world, the Yellow Emperor in China, the god Brahma and Vedic sages in India.
2. Their medical theories, formulated more or less coherently and assembled into a corpus, borrow their fundamental concepts from the speculations of contemporary philosophical schools regarding the universe, nature, man, the sociopolitical order, and so forth.
3. These medical traditions consider the body as a whole system of interrelated bodily functions, such as the circulation and transformation of humoral fluids, rather than mechanistically. They tend to explain physiological, pathogenic, or therapeutic processes in terms of sensible qualities, which they often express in contrasting pairs: hot/cold, dry/wet, active/passive, light/dark, and so on. These qualities, applied to different registers of reality—the parts of the body, mental or emotional dispositions, geography, and climate—are used to establish a system of correspondences between the microcosm and the macrocosm, integrating the individual as a psychosomatic entity into his spatial and temporal world. The world, society, and the unified entity of body and mind that is the human being are thus interrelated, reflecting one another in a rich and complex system of echoes, parallels, and metaphors.
4. Finally, these medical traditions tend to consider disease as a breakdown in the harmony of normal physiological functions. Curing disease thus means reestablishing harmony rather than rooting out a foreign invader. They share the same ideal of preventing illness through appropriate diet and lifestyle.

The Emergence of Medicine in India

A major source of Tibetan culture was India. It was there that Ayurveda developed as a learned medical tradition during the centuries prior to the birth of Christ. Its establishing texts include the Samhitas ascribed to Susruta and to Caraka, which are still in use today. These works be-

The root of diagnosis includes, left to right, visual observation, palpation, and inquiry (detail, pl. 13).

long to the normative literature of Brahmanism[1] that links the Ayurvedic medical tradition to the Vedas, India's earliest and most sacred scriptures (ca. 1500–700 B.C.E.). There are vast differences, however, between the essentially magico-religious therapy of the Vedas and even the earliest of the Ayurvedic Samhitas, which present, in an already systematized manner, knowledge and practices that can be regarded as truly medical. While we lack the historical documentation for this progressive development of the Indian medical traditions during the five or six centuries that must have separated the Vedic literature from the medical Samhitas, Buddhism played a role, possibly an important one, in that process.

Buddhism and Medicine

Buddhism displays affinities with medicine on many levels. As a doctrine and path of salvation, the eradication of disease becomes a metaphor for liberation from the endless cycle of rebirths. But the connections go deeper, with the problem of suffering being at the heart of Buddhist teachings from the very start. According to tradition, it was the young Prince Siddhartha's shocking first encounters with suffering in its most obvious biological manifestations—sickness, old age, and death—that incited the future Buddha to set out in search of an answer.

The answer became clear to him at the time of his Enlightenment, when the Buddha (566 or 563–486 or 483 B.C.E.) recognized the basic nature of all existence as suffering, comprehended its causes, and conceived the means by which one can be delivered and freed from the endless circle of suffering existence. The Four Noble Truths—defined as Suffering, the Cause of Suffering, the Removal of the Cause, and the Path leading to the Removal of the Cause—are characterized by the same simple, clear logic found in medical diagnosis. It is thus not surprising that very early on the Enlightened One acquired the designation of "supreme physician," and his teachings were seen as offering the only remedy radical enough to deliver the world's suffering beings—his "patients"—from their inherent predicament. Those who administered this remedy, members of the Buddhist monastic community, thus came to be regarded figuratively as attendants of the sick. Furthermore, Buddhists were never bound by the highly constraining rules of purity that governed the caste system at the base of Brahmanism. It was therefore easier for Buddhists to practice medicine, with its attendant risk of exposure to pollution through contact with the body and its substances. Although Buddhist monks were authorized to practice medicine within their own community, their treatment of lay people seems to have initially been greatly restricted, for two reasons: first, so as not to distract the monks from their primary objective of personal salvation; and second, to make sure that the alms they received from lay people not cease to be a free donation and become instead a form of payment for services rendered.

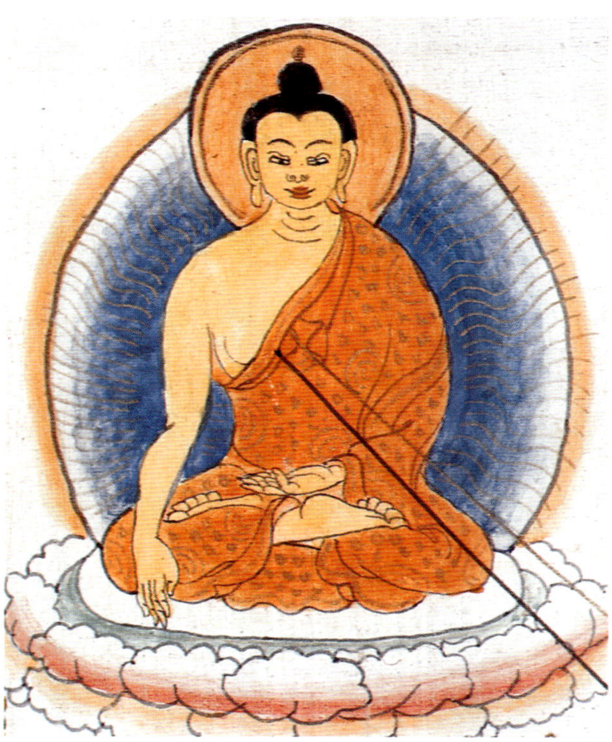

The Buddha Shakyamuni, a detail of plate 29 illustrating his compassion and spirituality being absorbed into the elixirs of rejuvenation.

Eventually this outlook changed. With the development of the Mahayana tradition in the first centuries of our era there came a new ideal—the bodhisattva—that offered a spiritual path for monks and

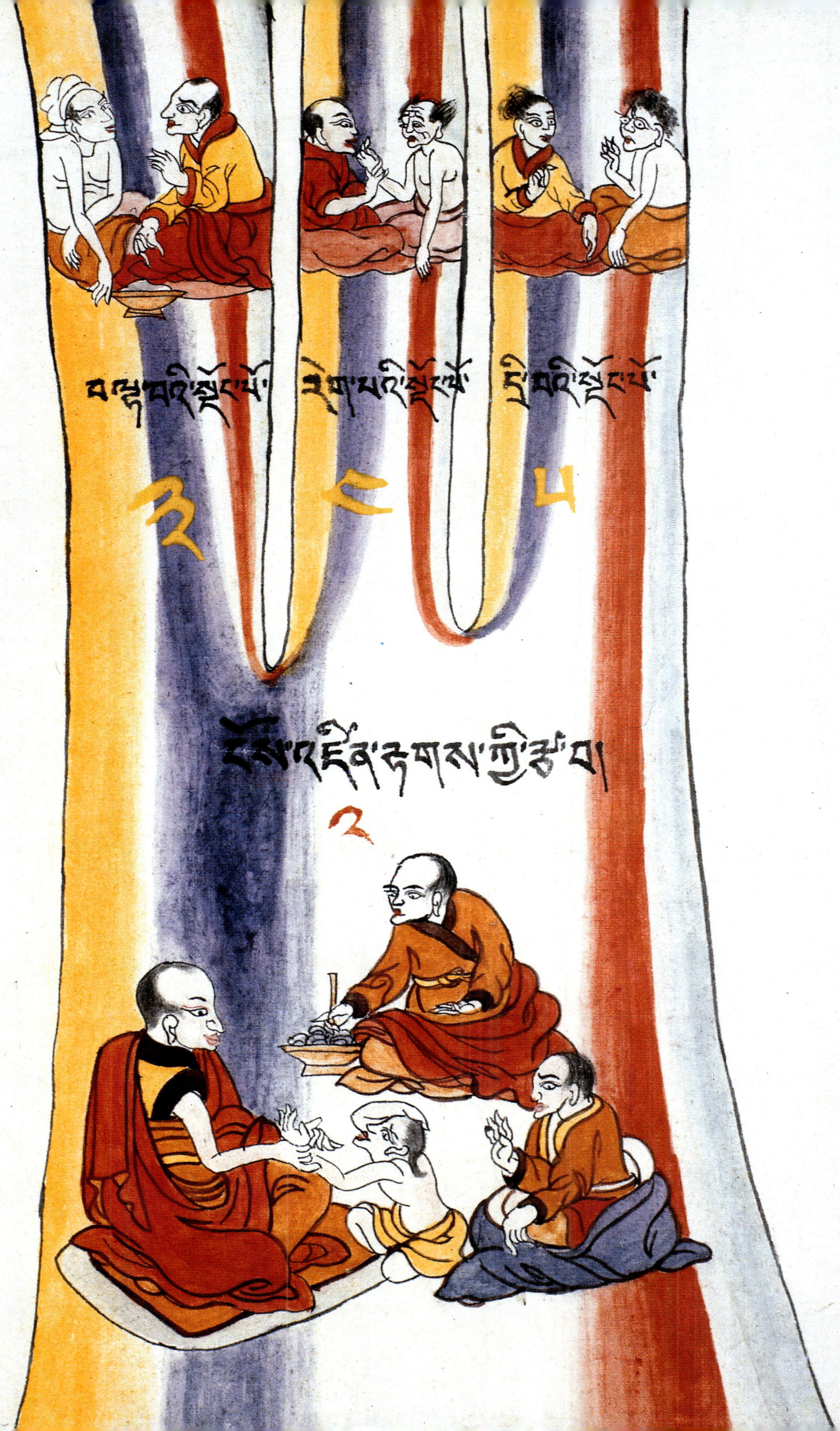

བལྟ་བའི་སྡོང་པོ་
རེག་པའི་སྡོང་པོ་
དྲི་བའི་སྡོང་པོ་
༣
༤
༥
ངོས་འཛིན་རྟགས་ཀྱི་རྩ་བ།
༢

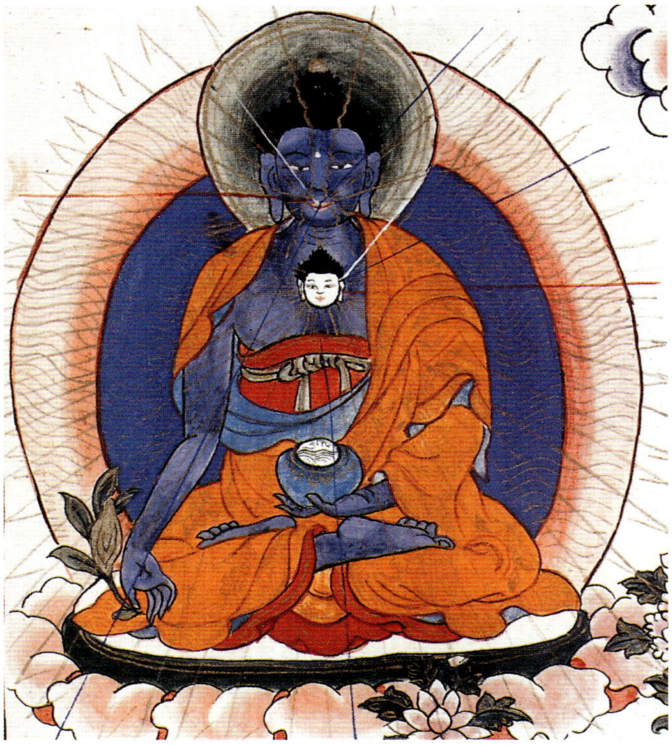

The Healing Buddha, originator of the teachings of Tibetan medicine. The rays emanating from his heart pacify all diseases and their causes: delusion, hatred, and desire (detail, pl. 2).

laity alike. For a bodhisattva, a "being devoted to enlightenment," the healing of the sick represented an opportunity to cultivate the perfections of compassion and generosity and also provided an effective means of conversion.[2] Medical practice became part of the curriculum of monastic studies, taking its place alongside the other four major sciences: the Buddhist "inner" science, grammar, epistemology, and the arts. Around the same time, the Buddhist pantheon was enriched with new figures possessing a specifically therapeutic function. One such figure, the Healing Buddha (Bhaisajyaguru) became the object of fervent worship in central Asia, in the Far East, and ultimately in Tibet (see the cover of this volume and plate 1). Buddhism's therapeutic aspects and the great renown of certain monks as healers undoubtedly contributed to its spread across Asia. But it was only in Tibet, as we discuss below, that a medical treatise was ascribed to the Healing Buddha. For the most part, it seems, the medicine practiced in Buddhist milieus relied on the same basic theory as the Hindu Ayurveda, with its central and fundamental notion of the three humors—wind, bile, and phlegm.

During the first millennium of the present era, the therapeutic traditions of India grew richer and more diverse. Conceptions of the body derived from the psycho-physiological techniques of yoga took their place alongside the classical tradition, as did, some time later, tantric teachings, both Hindu and Buddhist. A tradition of alchemy developed as well; its aim was to guarantee longevity or even immortality through the use of complex, often mercury-based, mineral preparations. And in the midst of all this, during the first half of the seventh century, a newly unified Tibet emerged as a formidable and expansionist military power in Asia.

The Development of Medicine in Tibet

Tibet's first great historical king, Songtsen Gampo (d. 649), conquered the neighboring kingdom of Shangshung in the west, made incursions into the southern Himalayas, and threatened the western confines of China. During the next two centuries, his dynastic successors extended this domain that had already reached imperial dimensions, bringing Tibet, the Land of Snows, into close contact with a number of prestigious civilizations. India, Kashmir, and Nepal, to the south, were still a repository of the high classical culture of the Gupta empire (320 to the end of the fifth century). In the west, influences from Iran and the more remote Mediterranean world intermingled with the Indian heritage, which was particularly present in the quite cosmopolitan northern oasis towns of the Silk Route. In the northeast and in the east, the influence and power of China's Tang empire (618 to 907) were also felt. Everywhere, Buddhism was a driving force of culture.

The Tibetans assimilated these new influences from neighboring civilizations with astonishing speed. A major one, of course, was Buddhism, which, together with its accompanying sciences, including medicine, was to leave a lasting mark on Tibet's history. The new state's administrative needs and its contacts from abroad led to the adoption of a system of writing. Tibetan tradition ascribes the new script to Songtsen Gampo, who is said to have commissioned its creation from an Indian prototype. Its adoption permitted the codification of a body of literature, and Tibetan historians record the seventh century as marking the birth of the Tibetan learned medical tradition, the Science of Healing.

Whereas previously Tibetan medicine had been confined to popular and magico-religious practices, during the following two centuries (the Tibetan dynastic period), medical developments reflected the cosmopolitan cultural influences of the period. Tibetan historians tell, for example, of several kings who summoned foreign physicians to the court from regions near and far: India, China, Iran, Kashmir, Nepal, the Turkic regions of Central Asia, and even "Byzantine lands." According to these sources, the teachings of these physicians were translated into Tibetan, some founding distinct lineages on Tibetan soil. A number of the practitioners mentioned in these accounts seem to have no concrete historical reality: for example, the evocation of "Galenos," a name that refers to Galen, the famous Greek physician of the second century of our era. Anachronistic though this reference is, it nevertheless testifies to the influence of Greek medicine that had reached the Tibetan empire via Iran and the Arabian conquest. Some documents of this period, as well as medical works still in use today, bear testimony to these various foreign influences. This is particularly true of some Indian and Chinese writings, to which the origin of Tibetan medicine is traditionally ascribed. The influence of Greek medicine can be detected, too, in certain rare borrowings and possibly in the Tibetan tradition of uroscopy.

The second wave of Buddhism's propagation in central Tibet dates from around the eleventh century, one hundred and fifty years after the fall of the Tibetan dynasty in 842, which brought about the territorial breakup of the kingdom. A period of intense religious, intellectual, and cultural activity had begun that would gradually transform the country in profound ways and shape its future. Whereas during the dynastic period Tibet's cultural contacts were marked by a wide cosmopolitanism, now the Tibetans turned mainly to India, receiving what was to be that country's final legacy of Buddhism and its related sciences before they disappeared from their native soil under the pressure of the Muslim conquests of the end of the twelfth century in the Ganges plain and two centuries later in Kashmir. Tibetan masters surrounded themselves with disciples, monks or lay tantric practitioners to whom they transmitted the teachings that they themselves had received. In the process they founded communities that in some cases evolved into distinct schools of religious thought and practice. Among them the Sakyapa school is of particular note, for it was given political power over Tibet during the Mongol protectorate of 1244 to 1368. Tibet was not to be reunified relatively permanently until the middle of the seventeenth century, under the aegis of the Gelugpa order and the Fifth Dalai Lama.

The Four Tantras (Gyushi)

The eleventh century also marked the start of a renaissance in Tibetan medical science. Several medical texts were translated from Sanskrit, eventually to be included in the the book of *Tangyur*, the Tibetan canonical collection of Buddhist commentaries and treatises. Along with the classical Indian medical tradition, Tibet adopted tantric conceptions of the body, notably

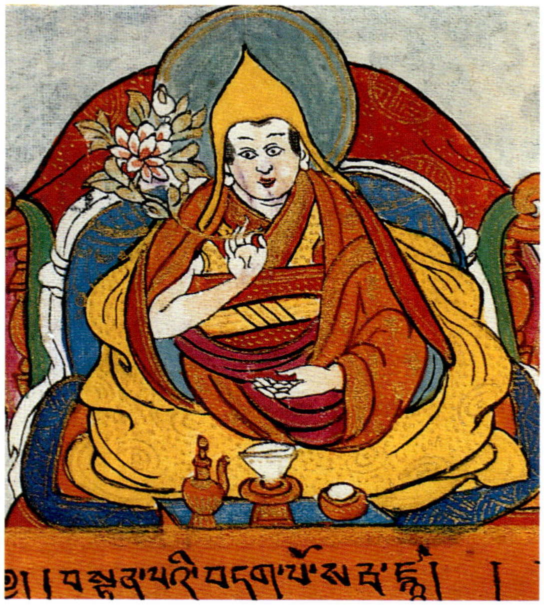

The Fifth Dalai Lama, who reigned during the classical period of Tibetan culture and medicine in the 17th century, when the paintings in this volume originated (detail, pl. 7).

those of the famous *Kalachakra Tantra,* as well as certain pharmacological techniques derived from the alchemical arts.[3] These borrowings were gradually adapted, enriched, and melded into a specifically Tibetan medical tradition closely allied with Buddhism. A rich literature developed: basic treatises and commentaries, pharmacopoeia, compilations of formulas for medicines, writings on the history of medicine, reference manuals devoted to specific diseases, diagnostic techniques, treatments, and so forth. Within this vast medical literature, the *Four Tantras* acquired particular preeminence and would eventually become the fundamental reference text used by Tibetan practitioners, nearly to the exclusion of all others. Many learned Tibetans accepted this treatise for what it claims to be: the word of the Healing Buddha. According to its colophon, the *Four Tantras* were translated from the Sanskrit into Tibetan in the eighth century and then hidden away by the famous master Padmasambhava, to be rediscovered during the second half of the eleventh century and finally completed and adapted to the local conditions of Tibet by Yuthog Yontan Gonpo the Younger in the twelfth century. This eminent origin and the transmission of the text as described in the colophon were ardently defended in the seventeenth century by the Fifth Dalai Lama and his last regent, Sangye Gyamtso. Nevertheless, some Tibetan scholars have gone so far as to deny the existence of a Sanskrit original and consider this text to be the work of a Tibetan author, observing quite correctly that it contains notions foreign to India, notably those appearing to be Chinese in origin. For the modern philologist, the *Four Tantras* in its present form cannot be considered to be the translation of a Sanskrit original. Rather, it appears to be the brilliant work of a Tibetan author, impossible to identify with certainty, who integrated the diverse foreign influences, predominantly those from India, into a coherent whole.

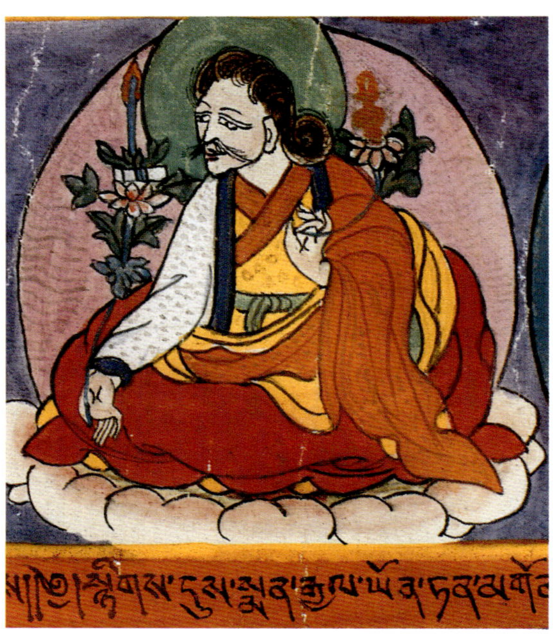

Yuthog Yontan Gonpo the Younger, "king among physicians" and the possible author of the *Four Tantras.* Here he is seated next to the "Protector of the Lives of Living Beings" within the illustration of the Tibetan medical-teaching lineage (detail, pl. 3).

For centuries, medical instruction in Tibet was carried out by individual masters who were independent of any particular institution. Texts, oral instruction, and practical techniques were passed down from master to disciple or from father to son in family lineages, often along with other medical and religious texts. Diplomas were not granted to mark the completion of studies, and the practice of medicine required no authorization from any civil or religious authority that might have imposed certain standards of theoretical knowledge and technical expertise. This method of transmission of medical knowledge and practices favored the emergence of various regional and family schools. Thus, after the fourteenth century, the Tibetan medical tradition split into two main schools, Chang and Zur. Differing only on minor questions such as the location of a few channels on the body (see plates 6–8), the identification of certain drugs and pharmaceutical formulas, and the interpretation of details in the *Four Tantras,* the two schools would later be reunited in the seventeenth century as part of the complete revamping of the teaching of Tibetan medicine initiated, as we shall see below, by Sangye Gyamtso. It is important to note, moreover, that this learned medicine with its written corpus was not the only medical resource. Instead it was an alternative or complement to other treatments, both popular and specialized, including folk medicine and religious practices, pilgrimages, shamanic cures, exorcisms, and healing rituals. Furthermore, Tibetan doctors did not form a homogeneous socioprofessional group; many practiced their trade alongside other, principally religious, activities.

The Fifth Dalai Lama and His Regent, Sangye Gyamtso

Efforts to bring about the political reunification of Tibet continued until the seventeenth century. These efforts, which enjoyed varying degrees of success, were often undertaken on behalf of noble families connected to Buddhist religious schools either under the direction of a foreign power—as was the case with the Sakyapas—or more or less autonomously. The political reunification of Tibet finally came about in 1642, under the aegis of the Fifth Dalai Lama and the Gelugpa religious order. It stands as a watershed event not only for the evolution of Tibetan culture as a whole but also for the field of medicine. The Dalai Lama, who had already shown interest in medical science in the course of his studies, undertook to promote its teaching and improve the quality of its practice. But it would be Sangye Gyamtso (1653–1705), his last regent and true spiritual heir, who would fulfill his vision. As a young man, the brilliant future regent had begun to study the *Four Tantras,* only to discover how confused the medical tradition had become over a number of theoretical and practical questions. And so he embarked on the ambitious enterprise of critically revising this text, drawing from a wide variety of written sources, either medical or of medical implication, as well as information obtained from various scholars. The regent's task, pursued alongside many other demanding literary and political activities, took nearly twenty years to complete. At the end of the seventeenth century it culminated in a revised edition of the *Four Tantras* and the composition of a brilliant commentary, the *Blue Beryl (Vaidurya ngonpo),* renowned to this day. The concern for didactic clarity that characterizes all of his medical works led the regent to create the series of seventy-nine paintings on canvas, forty of which are featured in the present book and the exhibition it accompanies. This series, referred to by N. D. Bolsokhoeva and K. M. Gerasimova as the *Atlas of Tibetan Medicine* and further described below

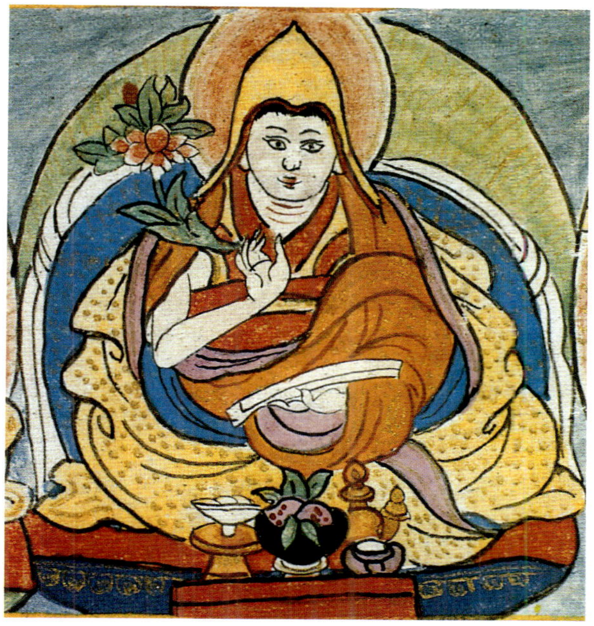

The Fifth Dalai Lama, seated here as part of the "Lineage of the Innermost Spirituality of Yuthokpa" (detail, pl. 5).

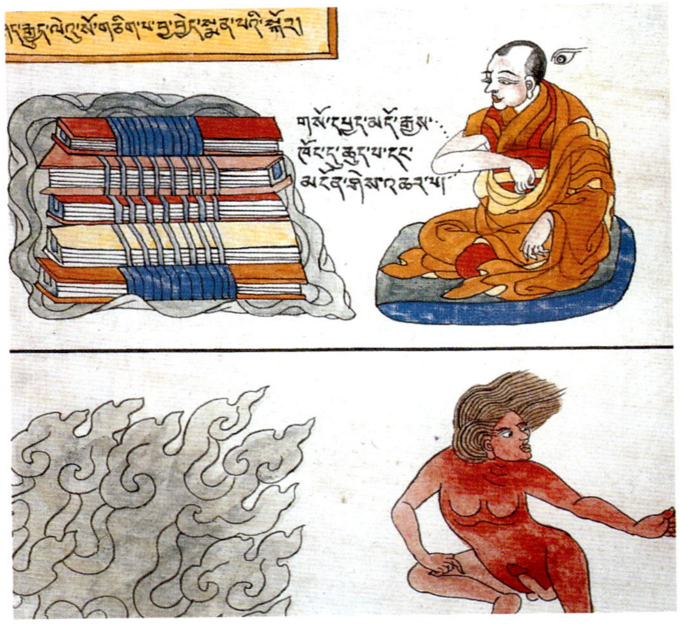

The qualities of a good physician include intelligence (illustrated in the study of the tantras), a caring attitude, the keeping of commitments, fitness of body, speech, and mind, perseverance, and knowing the ways of the world (detail, pl. 40). Below is an obstructing female demon of disease.

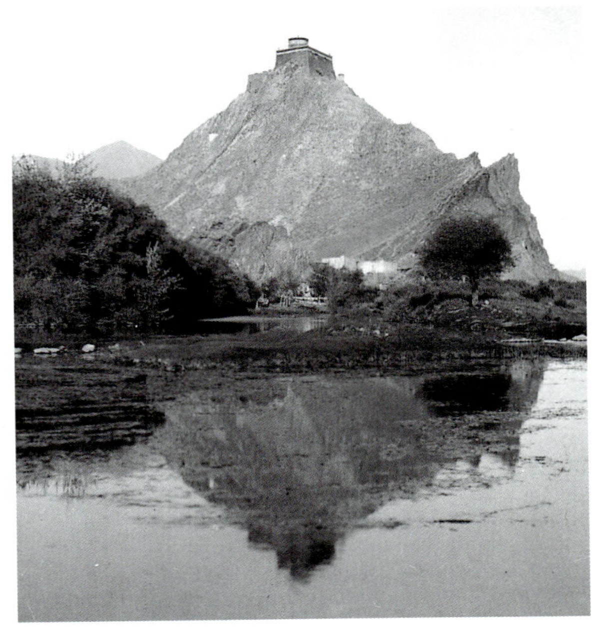

The medical college at Chagpori in 1932. Chagpori was founded in 1696 during the same period in which the paintings in this volume originated and destroyed in 1959. Most probably a set of the paintings was used there for study.

in my introduction to the catalogue section, illustrates the entire contents of the regent's commentary, including embryology, anatomy, physiology, *materia medica,* methods of diagnosis, and therapy.

At the time of the *Atlas* compiling, the country had just been reunified under a centralized authority and was thus entering into a process of cultural consolidation. The regent's ambition to codify and standardize Tibetan medical theory and practice led him to found, in 1696, the first college devoted specifically to medical instruction. The site of the college was Chagpori, the Iron Hill, facing the Potala Palace in Lhasa, which had once again become the capital of Tibet. Despite the specialized nature of the training given there, the administrative and academic organization of this institution on the whole continued to follow that of the Buddhist monastic colleges. Along with their training and medical activities such as collecting and processing medicinal plants, holding consultations, and treating patients, the residents devoted part of their time to activities of a religious nature: recitation of religious texts dedicated to the Healing Buddha, ritual consecration of remedies, and so forth. Those who wished also had the opportunity to further their study of astrology and the methods of calculation of the yearly calendar, many aspects of which were believed to have implications for medicine.

Chagpori acquired a prestige and influence worthy of the hopes the regent had invested in it at its inception. For two centuries it was the source of the physicians who administered to religious and secular leaders, both in central Tibet and in the eastern provinces, and even to members of the Chinese imperial court. During the sixteenth century, when the branch of Tibetan Buddhism practiced by the Gelugpa order had begun its massive propagation among the Mongols, Tibetan medical science followed in its wake. Practiced by monks for the most part, it spread beyond Mongolia proper to the Buryat Mongols of the Lake Baikal region in southern Siberia, reaching as far as the Kalmucks of the lower Volga. Chagpori provided a model for similar establishments not only in eastern Tibet (Kumbum, 1757; Labrang, 1784) and Beijing but also in Mongolia and among the Buryats.

Alongside these centers of institutionalized medical instruction with their systems of formal examinations, traditional Tibetan medicine continued to be transmitted unofficially, as in the past, by individual masters or within family lineages. The level of knowledge and practice among these individuals was thus quite varied.

At the end of the nineteenth century, Chagpori fell into decline until the Thirteenth Dalai Lama, following the example of the great Fifth, gave a new impetus to medical education. In 1916 he founded another medical college, the Mendzekhang, the School of Medicine and Astrology, in the very center of Lhasa, heralding the beginning of a new period of growth and renewal for Tibetan medical science. Under the direction of his personal physician Khyenrab Norbu (1883–1962), this new institution, open to monks and laity alike, enjoyed an influence to which most of the present famous practitioners can still attest. Khyenrab Norbu wrote a vast compilation of medicinal formulas now used as the standard reference both in Tibet and in the Tibetan community in exile. Like all areas of Tibetan culture, however, Tibetan medicine was profoundly affected by the wrenching political, economic, and social upheavals brought about by the Chinese domination of Tibet that began in 1950. The Chagpori college was destroyed during the Tibetan revolt of 1959, and indigenous traditional medicine as a whole was subjected to violent repression during the dark years of the Cultural Revolution. Nevertheless, in 1961, at the initiative of the current Dalai Lama, the Tibetan government-in-exile founded in Dharamsala, India, a center for traditional medical teaching and treatment, known today as the Tibetan Medical Institute. During these same years, individual physicians continued the tradition as refugees in various countries of the Himalayan region. In the last fifteen years or so, Tibetan medicine has aroused increasing interest worldwide. Its continued life among Tibetan refugees, its vitality in Tibetan-speaking regions of the Himalayas such as Ladakh, northern Nepal, and Bhutan, its resurgence in Chinese-controlled Tibet and even in Mongolia and Buryatia—all testify to a remarkable recovery.

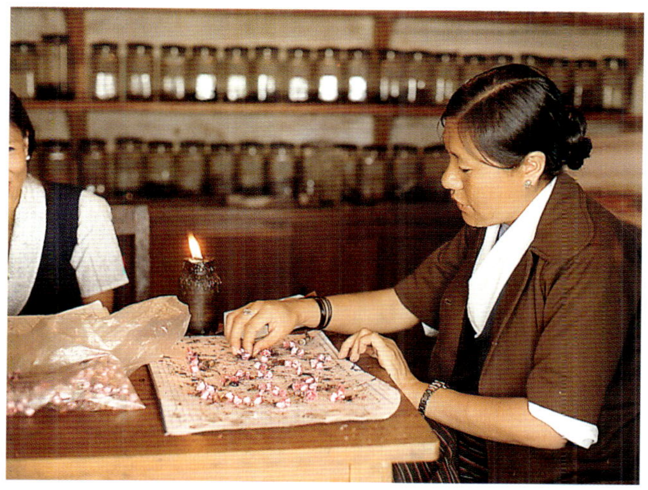

Tibetan doctor sorting "precious pills" in Dharamsala, India. These pills are composed of combinations of dozens of herbs, medicinal plants, and refined gemstones and minerals, each designed to enhance different aspects of the bodily system in order to restore a healthy balance.

Fernand Meyer

Translated from the French by Arthur Denner

Notes

1. The "normative literature of Brahmanism" refers not to Brahmanic literature but to the religious tradition, opposed to Buddhism, that links the Vedic period to late Hinduism.
2. The idea of conversion is here literally one of changing, "taming" the sentient beings.
3. The influence of the *Kalacakra Tantra* is particularly clear in the Tibetan medical speculations concerning the wheels of channels located at different levels of the body (see plate 6). As for the influence of Indian alchemy, it is manifest in the preparation of Precious Pills in which a great variety of metals and precious stones are compounded, as well as in the preparation of mercury-based remedies.

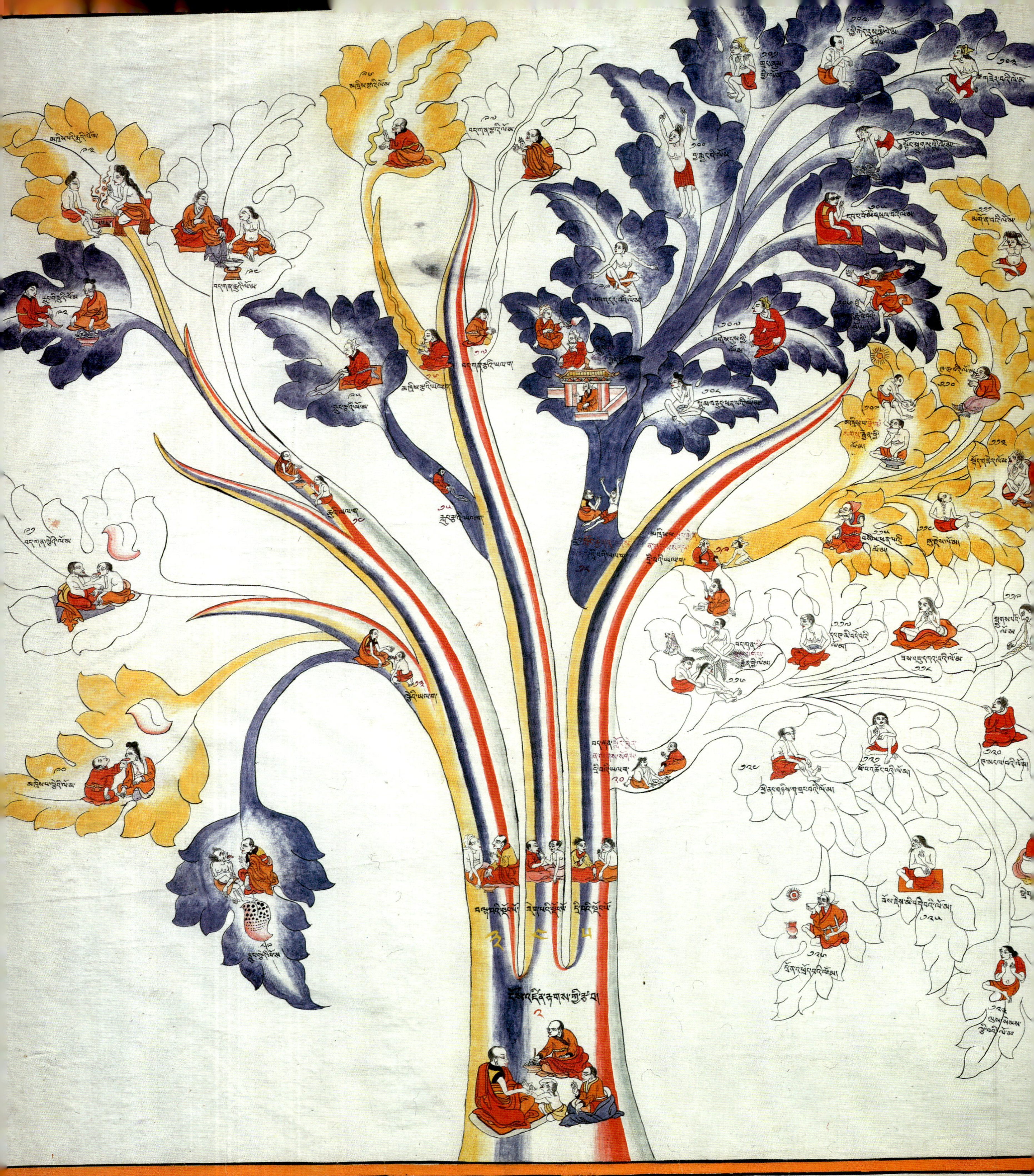

༣༧། །སྨན་བླའི་དགོངས་རྒྱན་རྒྱུད་བཞིའི་གསལ་བྱེད་བཻ་ཌཱུར་སྔོན་པོ་ལས་རྩ་རྒྱུད་ལེའུ་བཞི་པའི་དོན་འཛིན་རྟགས་ཀྱི་རྩ་བ་ལས། བལྟ་བ། རེག་པ། དྲི་བའི་སྡོང་པོ་གསུམ། དང་པོ་བལྟ་བའི་སྡོང་པོ་ལས། ལྕེ་དང་ཆུའི་ཡལ་ག་རེ་ལ་ལོ་འདབ་གསུམ་གསུམ་སྟེ་དྲུ
གཉིས་པ་རེག་པའི་སྡོང་པོ་ལས་རླུང་། མཁྲིས། བད་ཀན་གྱི་ཡལ་ག་གསུམ་ལས་ལོ་འདབ་ཀྱང་རེ། གསུམ་པ་དྲི་བའི་སྡོང་པོ་ལས་རླུང་མཁྲིས་བད་ཀན་གྱི་ཡལ་ག་གསུམ། རླུང་གི་ཡལ་ག་ལས་ལོ་འདབ་བཅུ་གཅིག། མཁྲིས་པའི་ཡལ་ག་ར་ལོ་འདབ་བདུན།། བད
ཀྱི་ཡལ་ག་ར་བཅུ་གཅིག་སྟེ་ཉེར་དགུ། དཔེ་བས་སྡོང་པོ་གསུམ། ཡལ་ག་བརྒྱད། ལོ་འདབ་སུམ་ཅུ་རྩ་བརྒྱད་ཡོད་ཚུལ་དུ་རྩ་བ་དམར་པོ། སྡོང་པོ་སེར་པོ། ཡལ་ག་སྔོ། ལོ་མ་སྔག་ཚའི་ཨཀྲི་རི་སྦྲངས་དང་བཅས་པ་བཀོད་པ་སྟེ་ཁྲིས་ཆ་གསུམ་པའོ།།

The Atlas of Tibetan Medicine

Treasures from the History Museum of Buryatia

It is the time of Stalin's terror in the mid-1930s. Churches, temples, and Buddhist monasteries (datsans) *are being razed throughout the Soviet Union as the campaign against religion is carried out. The Atsagat Datsan in eastern Siberia (Transbaikalia) has been visited by Z. Zhabon, an official of the Society of the Militant Godless (the anti-religious arm of the Communist party), who spends all night talking to one of the resident lamas. Zhabon has learned of the existence of the* Atlas of Tibetan Medicine, *a rare and beautiful group of Buddhist* thangkas, *and he tells the lama that he wants them for the museum in Ulan-Ude, Buryatia. The lama is suspicious, but Zhabon is a skilled negotiator; as dawn approaches the lama climbs the stairs to the attic where the paintings have been hidden and hands them over to Zhabon.*[1] *Less than a year later, the Atsagat monastery is destroyed. True to his word, however, Zhabon delivers the* Atlas *safely to the museum in Ulan-Ude.*

For the past six decades, the *Atlas* paintings have been kept in the safety to which they were entrusted by a Buddhist lama whose name is now lost to history: the safety of the History Museum of Buryatia. Here they have been carefully protected in the eighteenth-century museum building that is called the Hodigitriya, originally a Russian Orthodox cathedral. The paintings first came to the attention of scholars in 1958. K. M. Gerasimova had become aware of their existence, and she assisted in making them available to the pharmacologist A. F. Gammerman and the Tibetologist A. V. Semicov as source material for the book they were working on, a Tibetan-Latin-Russian dictionary of Tibetan medicine. This work consequently incorporates the names of 540 medicinal herbs and plants as drawn and identified in the *Atlas.* In 1968 under the leadership of P. B. Baldanzhapov, a group of Buryat scholars and lamas began the intensive study of the series and its relation to Tibetan medical practices in Buryatia. The present volume accompanies the first public exhibition of these paintings.

The Tree of Diagnosis (detail, pl. 13), illustrating how Tibetan physicians diagnose illness when the three humors are imbalanced. In the right trunk the method of questioning is illustrated, with the physician asking questions about symptoms, location of the pain, and which foods help or harm the patient.

How did this priceless artifact—the outline of an entire system of medical diagnosis and treatment—find its way from Tibet to Buryatia? There are two stories that answer this question. The first is that the *Atlas* was acquired between 1905 and 1907 by famed Buryat scholar Bazar Baradin of Aginsk during his journey to Labrang (Amdo Province), the birthplace of the Dalai Lama.[2] The second version has the history of the *Atlas* and its tortuous journey beginning in the late nineteenth century with a Buryat lama and physician, Shirab Sunuev (1860–1930; also of Aginsk), who made an extraordinary trek across the mountains to bring the scrolls from Tibet to Transbaikalia. Specifically, the *Atlas* was brought to the Tsugol Datsan in the Transbaikal region from the Medical College of Serkhog, located in northeastern Tibet, where Sunuev had studied medicine for ten years. It is said that the paintings were kept at Tsugol until about 1926, when, at the request of the famous Buryat lama Agvan Dorzhiev (1840–1938) they were moved to the Medical College of Atsagat by Danzan Norboyev, who was at that time effectively acting as Dorzhiev's deputy and serving as the unofficial spiritual representative of the Dalai Lama.[3] Ten years later the paintings were deposited in the Museum of Atheism (now

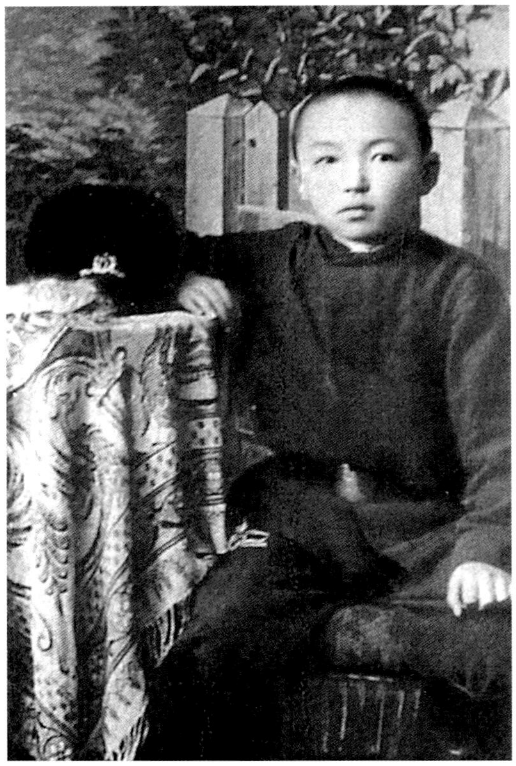

Bazar Baradin as a child. Baradin was a prominent figure in the Buddhist community in Buryatia; he attempted to reconcile Buddhism and Bolshevism, but was eventually shot in the Stalinist purges in 1936.

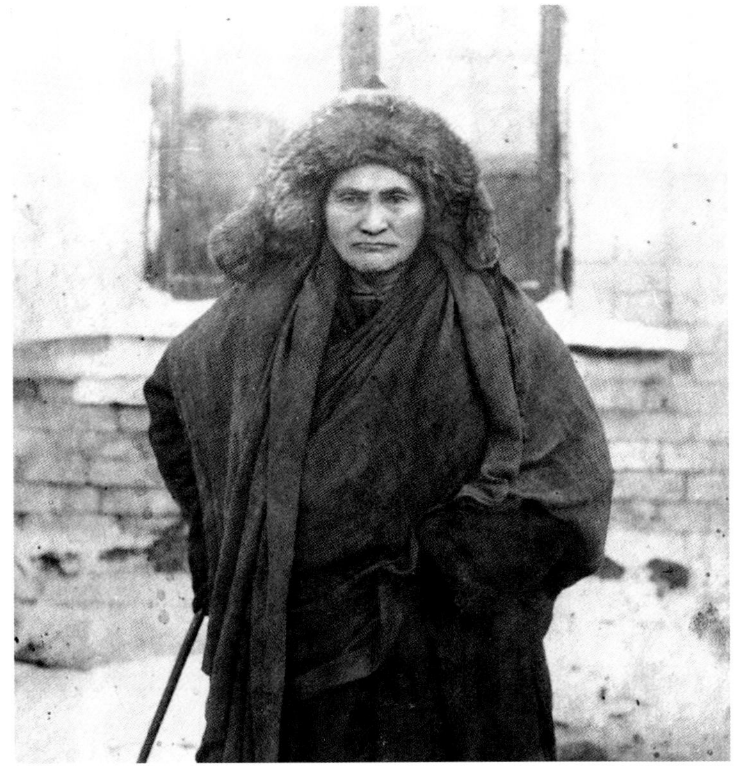

Agvan Dorzhiev, 1928. Dorzhiev is thought to have commissioned the paintings in this volume and the exhibition. Dorzhiev was born in Buryatia and became a chief advisor and teacher of the Thirteenth Dalai Lama.

The Aginsk (sMan-pa) Datsan, where a medical college was opened in 1884. This datsan is reported to have been rebuilt, as part of the revival of Buddhism in Russia.

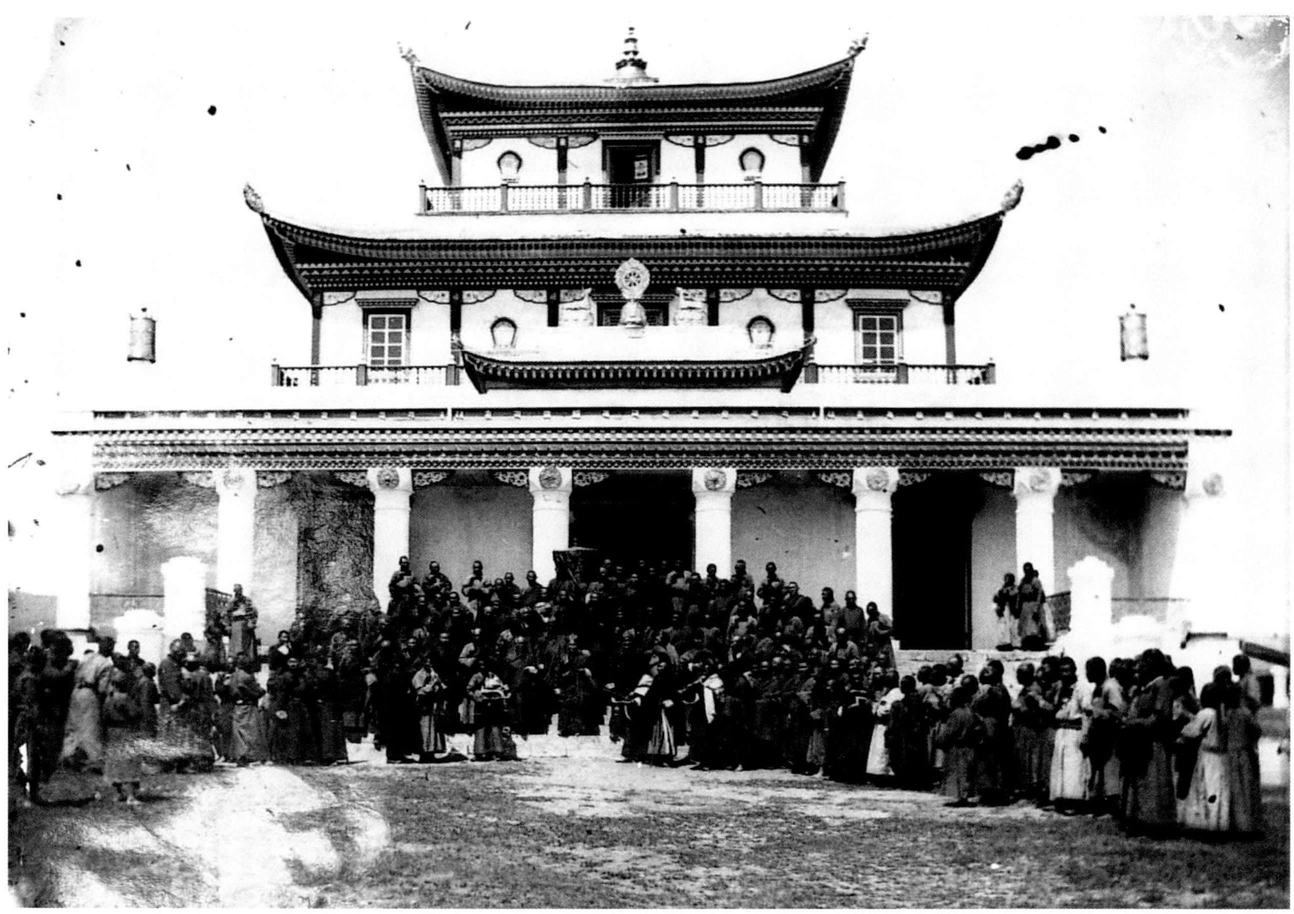

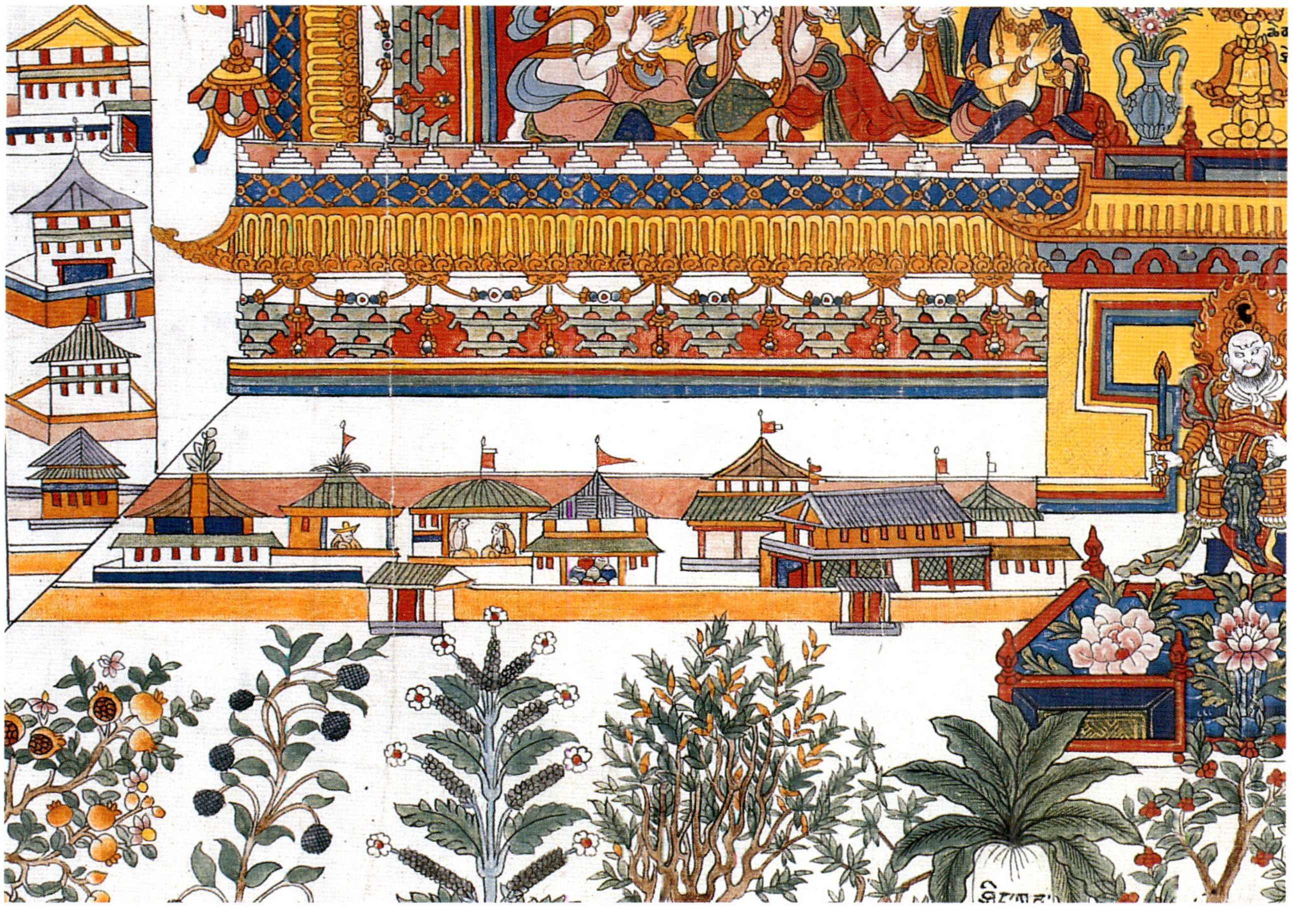

Buildings of the outer area of Sudarsana, the City of Irresistible Beauty in which the Healing Buddha originally gave the medical teachings (detail, pl. 1).

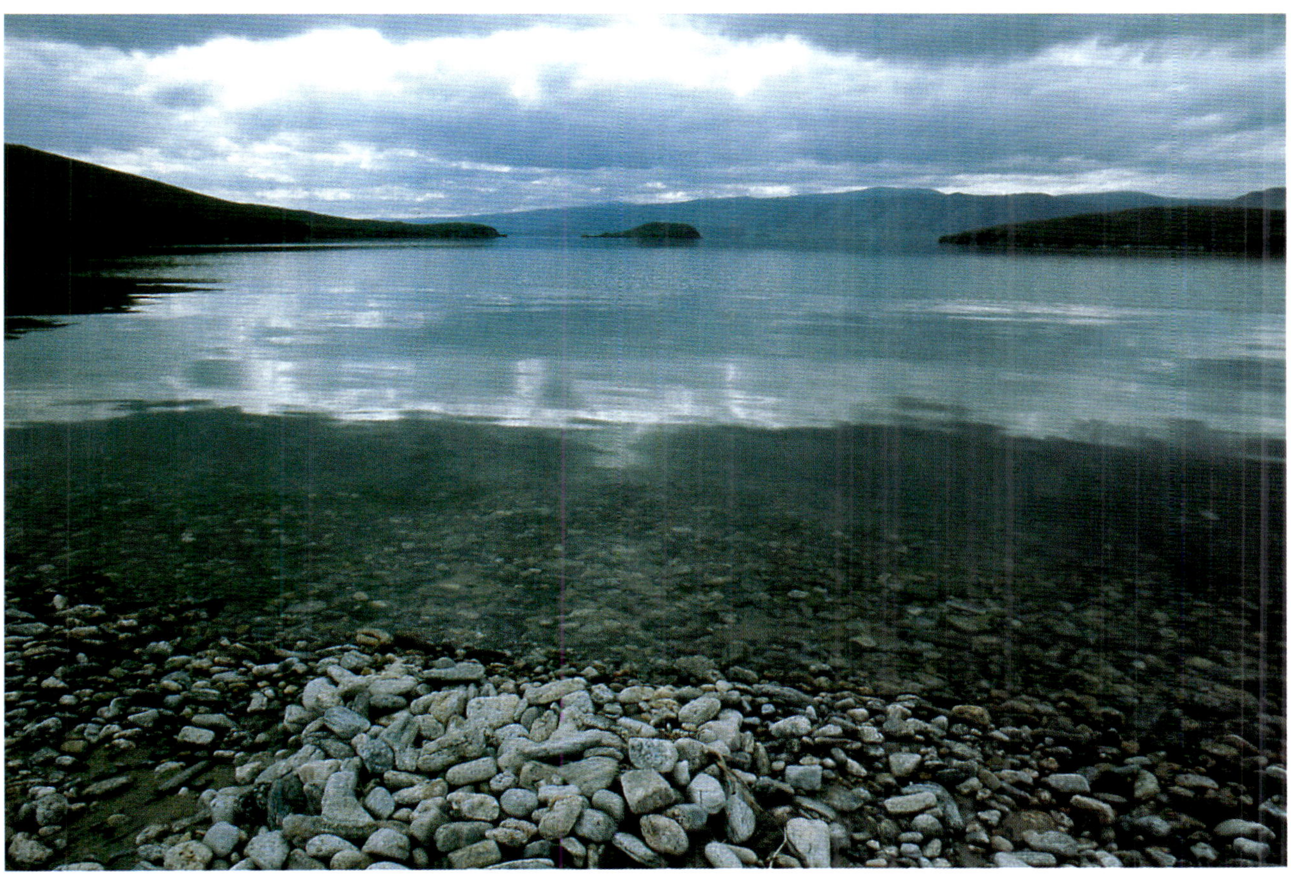

Lake Baikal, Buryatia, a prominent feature of the area in which Buddhism has been traditionally practiced in Russia. The deepest freshwater lake in the world, it is home to ancient species now extinct elsewhere, and is considered sacred by many of the indigenous peoples of Siberia.

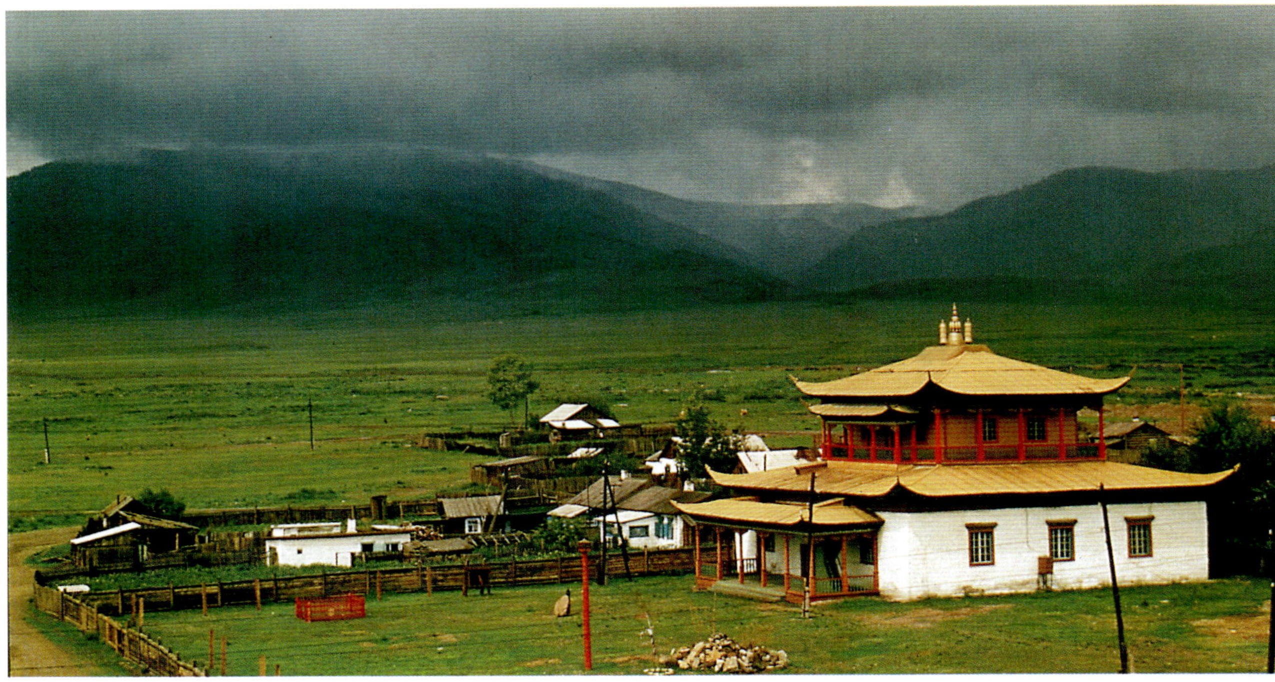

The Gusinoyozerso Datsan in Buryatia, one of the oldest monasteries in Russia. Established in 1741, it is reported to have been closed in 1930 during the Stalinist campaign against religion, but appears to have been rebuilt.

the History Museum of Buryatia) by Z. Zhabon, who was the chief curator of the archive from 1952 to 1970.[4]

Whoever made the journey with the *Atlas,* he no doubt had a difficult trip. At that time Tibet was closed to foreigners by the Qing government of China and the Lhasa troops, though natives of the countries of Asia who professed Buddhism were allowed to enter Lhasa for a brief visit.[5] Making a pilgrimage to Tibet involved delicate political negotiations and treacherous travel conditions: extreme heat and cold, and a lack of water and food.

Buddhism in Russia

Before entering into an examination of the paintings themselves and the medical treatises they illustrate, it will be illuminating for the Western reader to describe the setting of the museum from which they now come. Located in the central part of the Asian continent, the Buryat Republic is situated in eastern Siberia between Lake Baikal, the deepest freshwater lake in the world, and Mongolia. Lake Baikal is truly one of Russia's greatest natural treasures.

The Buryats are the indigenous ethnic group for whom the Buryat Republic was named and who, from ancient times, settled the land to the west and east of the sacred Lake Baikal. Related to the Mongols through language, physical characteristics, and cultural tradition, they are one of the largest among the so-called native peoples of eastern Siberia, with a population of 422,000. Until the early twentieth century, they were nomadic cattle herders on the dry steppes. The most vivid features of the Buryats' material culture were the complex and beautiful decoration of both horse and rider, the round felt yurt with its unique interior, and the elaborate and colorful dress of the men and women, further ornamented with a lavish use of silver.

Buddhism arrived in Buryatia from Tibet via Mongolia around the mid-seventeenth century, and by the end of the eighteenth had spread to southern and eastern Buryatia (the Transbaikal region). The official date of its recognition is considered to be 1741, when the Empress Elizaveta Petrovna legalized the existence of 11 datsans and the 150 lamas in them. Buryatia became the seat of the northernmost branch of the central Asian variation of Mahayana Buddhism that developed in Tibet. The Gelugpa school of Tibetan Buddhism (founded by the prominent reformer Tsong Khapa, 1357–1419) had the most followers in the Transbaikal area.

The Buryat datsans were established on auspicious sites, in keeping with Buddhist tradition. The blue peaks of the Buryat mountains were their backdrop, and the view must have been spectacular: rivers and smooth lakes, and the expansive steppes as far as the eye could see. The remoteness and isolation of the datsans emphasized the Buddhists' renunciation of everything worldly and the datsans' connection with the heavenly.

Important centers of culture and education, datsans (the term *datsan* is derived from Tibetan *dratsang,* meaning monastic college) also sometimes housed schools and clinics of Tibetan medicine. The earliest were founded in the early eighteenth century (Sartulsk Datsan was founded in 1707, Tsongol in 1730, and Gusinoyozerso in 1741). Prior to the October Revolution, there were forty-seven functioning datsans and dugans (prayer houses) with an official monastic population of sixteen thousand. The Tsugol Datsan, dating from 1826, was built on the gentle south slope of a hill rising above the broad washes of the mouth of the river Onon, and beginning in 1869, medicine was taught there. The teaching was based on the system developed by the medical faculty of the Labrang monastery. Our limited information on this subject derives from the oral traditions of Buryat lamas or laypeople. It is known that Tuguldurov of the Tsugol Datsan had invited the Mongolian lama Chos sMan-rams-pa, who took on the responsibility of teaching Tibetan medical practices to the lamas there. After his death the teachings were interrupted until 1899, when they were reestablished under the guidance of the Buryat scholar Darma Biliktuyev. After the medical school was established at the Tsugol Datsan, the teachings were introduced at several other datsans in the area. The largest was at Atsagat, which had almost sixty students;

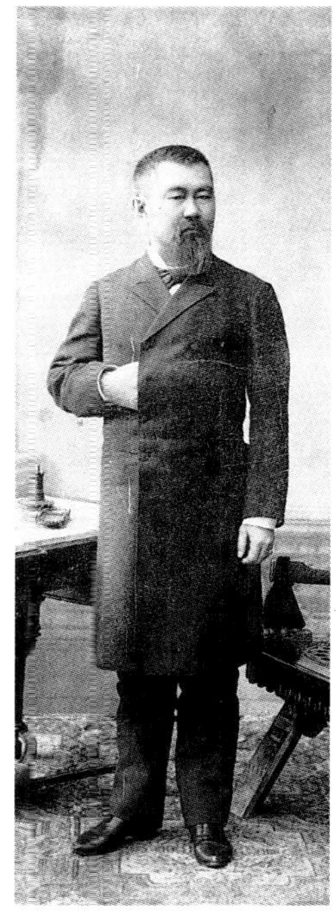

Piotr Badmayev (1856–1919), one of the most important figures in the expansion of Tibetan Buddhist medical doctrines. A Buryat doctor of Tibetan medicine, Badmayev established a flourishing practice of Tibetan medicine in Saint Petersburg.

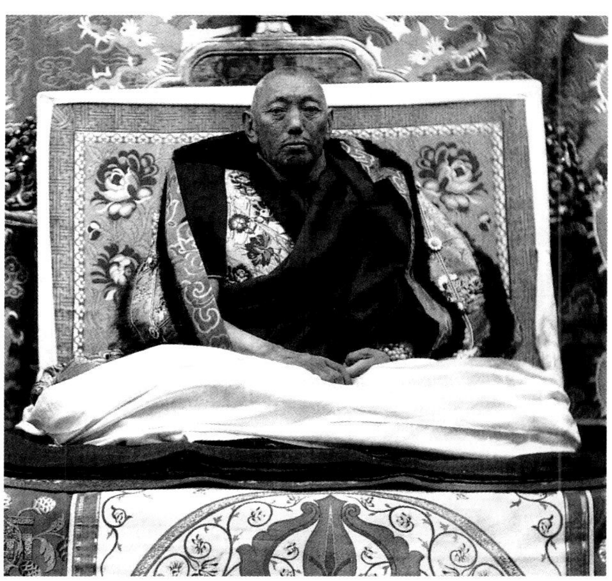

The Thirteenth Dalai Lama Tubten Gyatso (1876–1933), on his throne in Lhasa, Tibet.

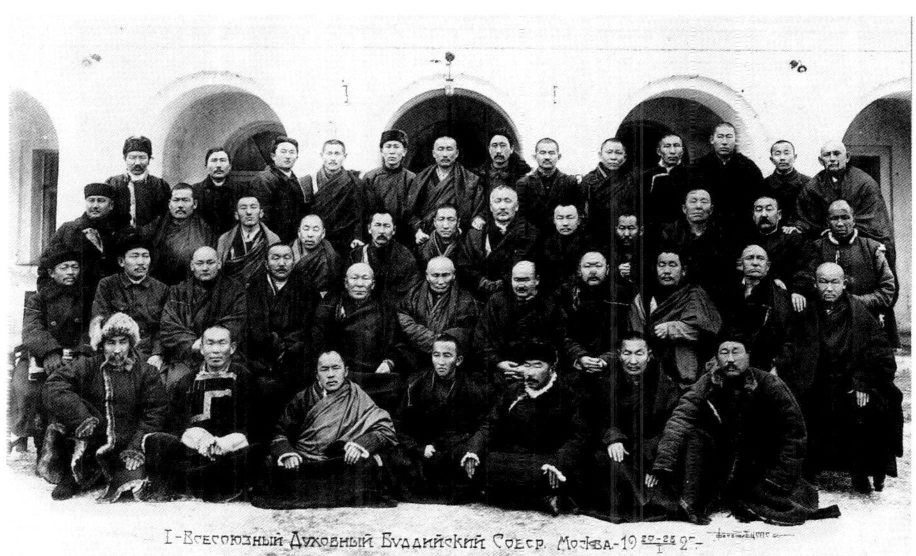

Agvan Dorzhiev (center) at the first All-Russian Buddhist Congress meeting in Moscow, January 20–29, 1927.

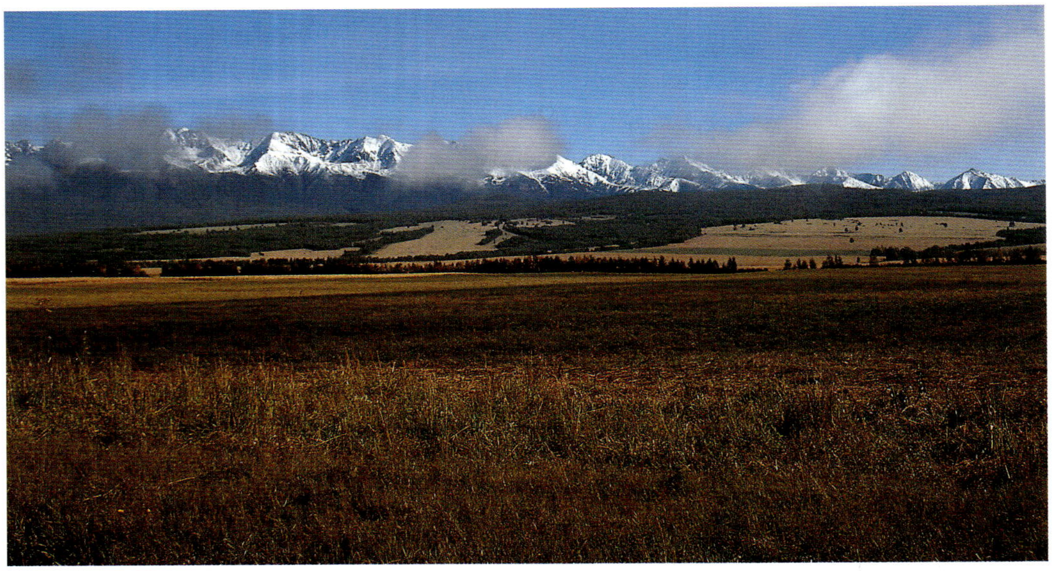

at the Aginsk Datsan around the same number of doctors of Tibetan medicine were practicing. The Atsagat Datsan broke away from the Ana Datsan in 1825 and in 1877 moved to a new location. With the direct involvement of Agvan Dorzhiev, construction of a school of Tibetan medicine with an infirmary began in 1908 and the school, located on a site chosen for its healing waters, was opened in 1913.

The Tunka Valley in the Sayan Mountains, Buryatia, where vast expanses of grassy steppe extend to the base of the glacier-covered peaks.

One of the most important figures in the expansion of Tibetan Buddhist medical doctrines was Piotr Aleksandrovich (Zhamtsaran) Badmayev (1856–1920), born in Aginsk (Chita region). An orientalist and political figure, Badmayev was primarily committed to the practice and scientific study of Tibetan medicine, appearing to have been initiated by his elder brother, Tsultim Badmayev, a Buddhist lama and doctor of Tibetan medicine. Piotr Aleksandrovich was highly educated and well connected, with patients who were ministers and senators. Czar Nicholas II (1868–1918) became greatly interested in the methods of treatment and remedies of the Tibetan medical system, and Badmayev, a frequent visitor to the palace, became the family's personal physician. He also maintained a school in Saint Petersburg and supported students from his homeland with scholarships to the School of Oriental Studies at Saint Petersburg University. One such

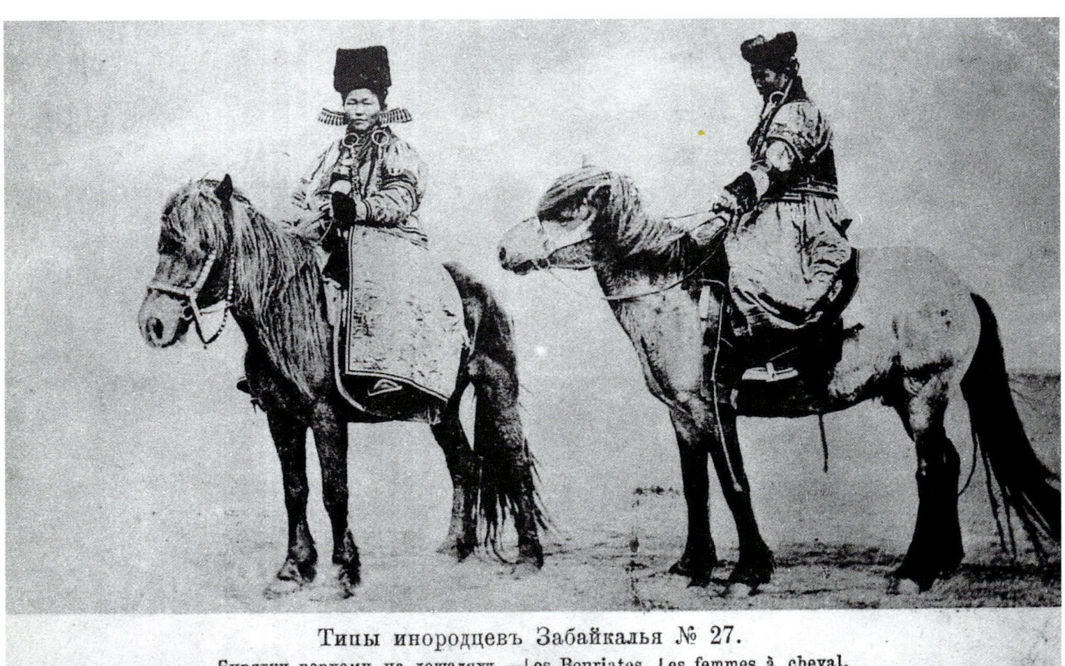
Типы инородцевъ Забайкалья № 27.
Бурятки верхами на лошадяхъ.—Les Bouriates. Les femmes à cheval.

Buryats in traditional dress, possibly 1890s. The Buryats began to wear Russian-style clothes in the early part of the twentieth century.

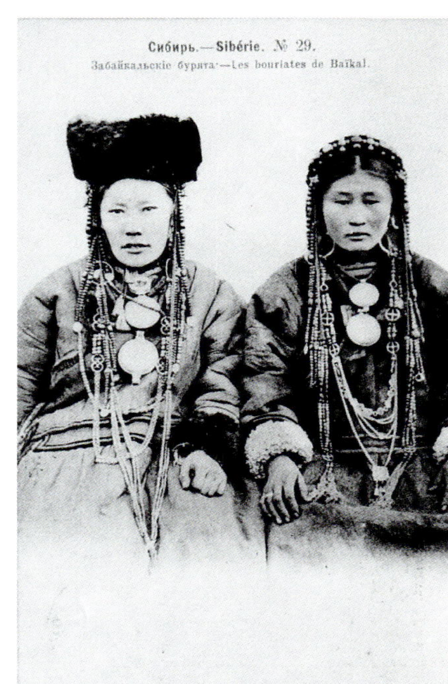
Сибирь.—Sibérie. № 29.
Забайкальскіе буряты.—Les bouriates de Baïkal.

Buryat women traditionally wore earrings and necklaces inscribed with Tibetan prayers.

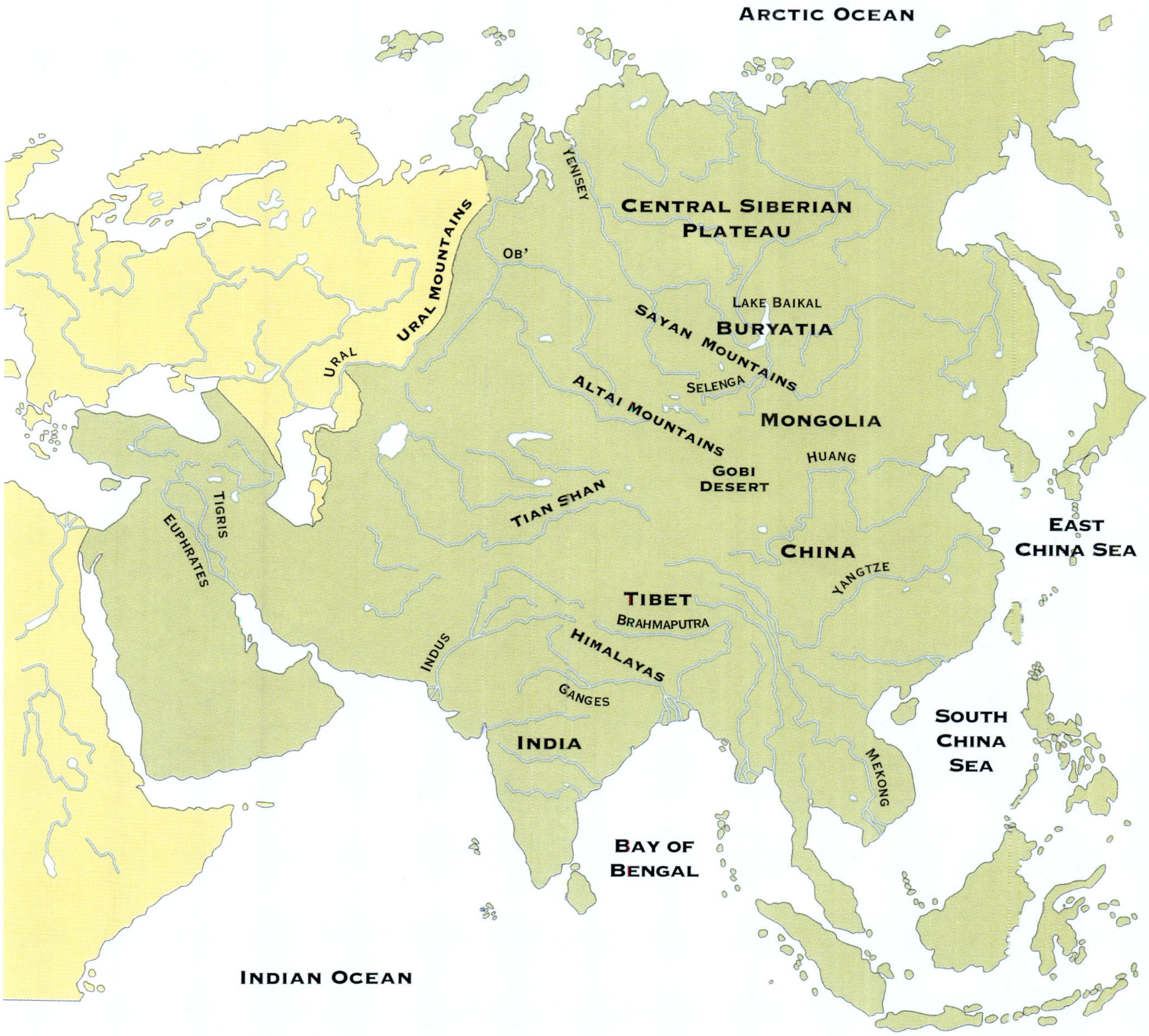

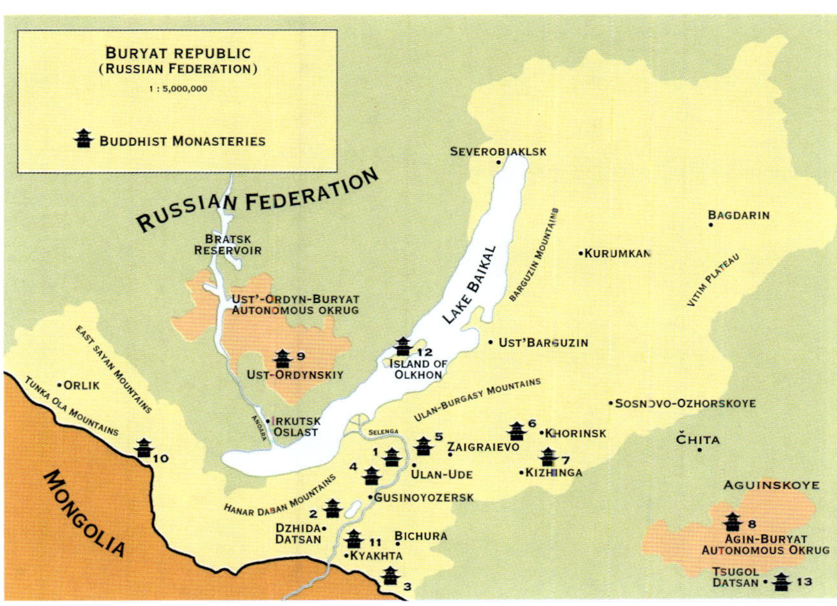

Selected Buddhist Monasteries of Buryatia

Names and Years of Establishment

1. *Ivolga Datsan*	1949
2. *Gusinoyozerso Datsan*	1741
3. *Tsongol Datsan*	1730
4. *Yangazhin Datsan*	1830
5. *Atsagat Datsan*	1825–31
6. *Ana Datsan*	1775–95
7. *Eguita Datsan*	1824–26
8. *Aga Datsan*	1811–16
9. *Alar Datsan*	1814
10. *Kirensk Datsan*	1817
11. *Dzhida Datsan*	1749
12. *Kharatsa Datsan*	1918
13. *Tsugol Datsan*	1826

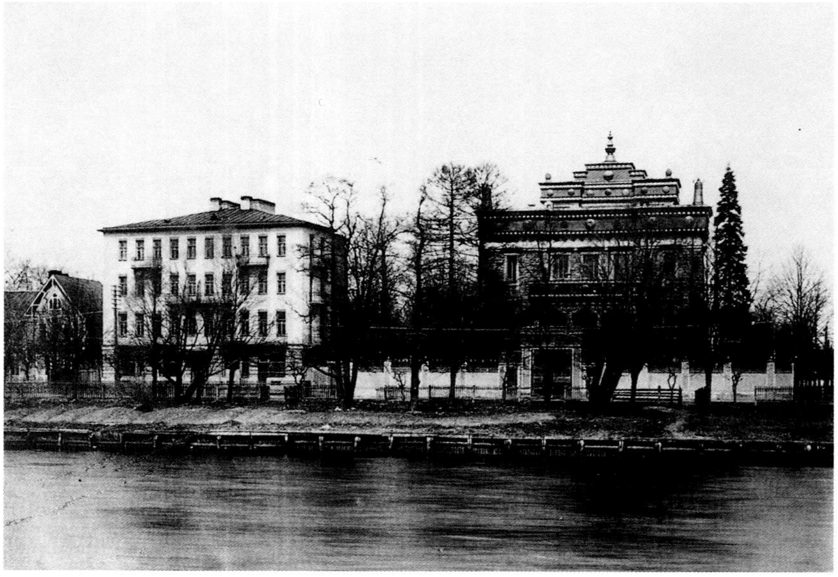

The Saint Petersburg Buddhist temple founded by Agvan Dorzhiev in 1909 and consecrated in 1915. The building still stands.

scholarship was awarded to the Buryat student G. Tshybikov, who later became a well-known scholar in the field of Tibetan and Mongolian studies. With the support of the Russian Imperial Geographical Society, Tshybikov organized a pilgrimage to Tibet, publishing a book on the subject of his travels in 1919.

Tibet has long been near and dear to all Buryat Buddhists. They say prayers in the Tibetan language, give their children Tibetan names, and dream of a pilgrimage to Tibet. Though until recently the trip was incredibly difficult, most Buryat lamas traveled to Tibet to obtain an authentic Buddhist education. One of these was the aforementioned Shirab Sunuev, whose former students have described how he brought the paintings with him to Buryatia, where Buddhist medical students at the Tsugol Datsan used them as visual aids in the study of the fundamentals of medicine.[6]

Agvan Dorzhiev, founder of the medical college at the Atsagat Datsan, to which the paintings were transferred, was one of the most prominent Buryat Buddhist figures of the turn of the century. Considering his importance in the second version of our story, a look at his biography is warranted.

Dorzhiev was born in the Khara-Shibiri Khorin Steppe Duma near the Atsagat Datsan. He was a scribe in the office of the Khorinsk Steppe Duma, a family man who lived as a successful secular official. Suddenly, his life changed drastically. The lama Namanai-Gegen took him as a student, ordained him as a monk, and sent him incognito "under the name of a Mongol" to study in the famous Gomang College at the Drepung monastery just west of Lhasa.[7]

By the age of thirty-five, Dorzhiev had received a degree in philosophy, known as the *tsannid khenpo lharamba.* He numbered among seven of the best scholars in the retinue of the Thirteenth Dalai Lama, teaching him Buddhist philosophy and literature. His status as mentor of the Dalai Lama enabled him to become a prominent advisor and major figure in the Tibetan theocratic government. In 1898, he went to China, Russia, and France to learn about their governmental structures and lifestyles. Upon returning to Tibet he was elevated to the third highest of the senior *khambo* with the right to speak on all matters of policy and faith.[8]

After the October Revolution and through the thirties, a reform movement arose among the lamas of Buryatia, headed by Dorzhiev and Bazar Baradin. The movement advocated cleansing the ancient, "pure" Buddhism from superstition and charlatanism, renouncing the parasitic way of life, and recognizing the Soviet government and the need to be occupied with productive labor. Dorzhiev's entire purpose was to adapt Buddhism to socialism and preserve Buddhism in the new Soviet society. As a result, the contemporary Buryat Buddhist church was founded.

Perhaps in reaction to the reform movement, beginning in 1928, in the cities and villages of Buryatia, antireligious propaganda grew more active. In 1929, the Society of the Militant Godless was formed; within a year it officially numbered twelve thousand members. The press, book publishing industry, cultural institutes, ethnographic museums, and so on were enlisted in the campaign.[9] Dorzhiev's archives show that he was untiring in his struggle to preserve Buddhism in Russia.[10]

Agvan Dorzhiev succeeded in obtaining the consent of Czar Nicholas II to build a Buddhist temple in Saint Petersburg, hoping that it could become a kind of representation of the Dalai Lama in Russia. Yet by 1935, a third of the datsans were empty due to the absence of lamas, although officially not a single datsan had been closed. In 1936, the Soviet Union was given a constitution whose statutes proclaimed the existence of a perfect democracy, which flagrantly misrepresented the lawlessness of the time. During Stalin's reign, one of the "most large-scale, terrifying, and mysterious phenomena of the twentieth century,"[11] nearly all the datsans were shut down and the lamas were exiled, sent to work camps, or executed. In 1937 the Atsagat Datsan was destroyed.

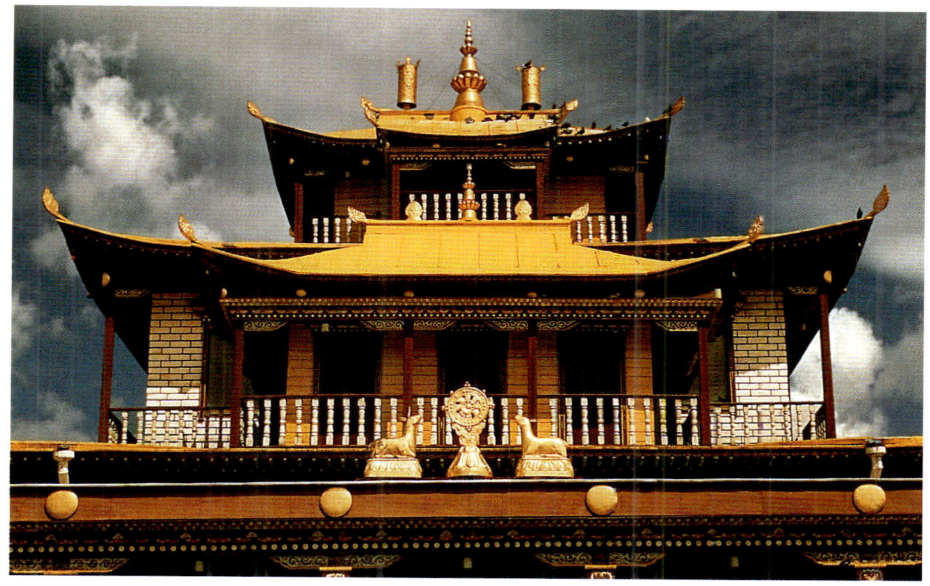

The Ivolga Datsan in Buryatia. The Fourteenth Dalai Lama visited here in 1979 during his first visit to Russia.

During this period, Dorzhiev retreated to the Saint Petersburg temple, then returned to Buryatia in 1938 and settled in the village of Atsagat, where he was arrested in Stalin's roundup of religious figures. According to one story, he died in prison in Ulan-Ude; according to another, he was released due to physical incapacitation and died on the road home to Atsagat.[12]

Within this very difficult environment, scholars, museum workers, and enthusiasts of the cause collected Buddhist objects for the museum. In cars, on horses, and on their own backs, they carried the treasures out of the ruins of the datsans, and stored what they could in the Hodigitriya Cathedral and on its grounds. The Museum of Religion and Atheism was opened on the first floor, but was soon closed.[13] It eventually became the M. N. Khangalov History Museum of Buryatia. As L. N. Gumilev has noted, "for a long time the Buryat monasteries preserved paintings or copies of works lost in Tibet itself, Khotan, and China, and artifacts that had been the objects of archeological digs in India. Here, as in a drop of water, are reflected the heavens, the traces preserved of the ancient culture of central Asia, and the life that disappeared many centuries ago."[14]

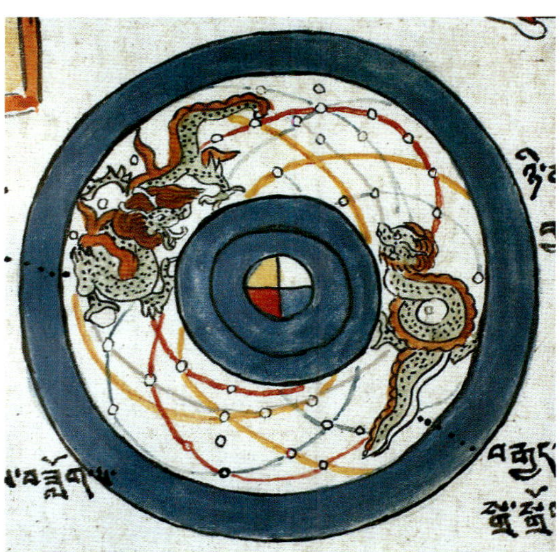

The solar system after the summer solstice (detail, pl. 21), illustrating proper conduct, which from the Tibetan viewpoint is one remedy for disease; each season has specific requirements.

Yet Buddhism by no means disappeared in Russia. Around 1946 the Ivolga Datsan was built not far from Ulan-Ude to commemorate the war efforts of Buryat Buddhists, and the slow and difficult process of the rebirth of Russian Buddhism began. Activities initiated around 1989 and 1990 may be said to constitute a revival, and some of the lamas have returned from the cities to their homelands in order to reopen datsans. In 1992 Atsagat Datsan was rebuilt.

The *Atlas of Tibetan Medicine:* A Vision of the Whole

The *Atlas of Tibetan Medicine* in the historical museum's archives[15] consists of seventy-six paintings, although they are numbered through seventy-seven (forty of these have been selected by Fernand Meyer to appear in this exhibition and book).[16] Each painting has a different number of drawings (from 90 to 274); altogether there are approximately 10,000, which are stunning in artistry of execution and freshness of color. Captions in Tibetan under each drawing in the *Atlas* are excerpted from the *Four Tantras* and the *Lapis Lazuli* [the *Lapis Lazuli* is synonymous with the document referred to elsewhere in this volume as the *Blue Beryl*—Ed.]. When one considers the series as a whole, it quickly becomes obvious that it would be a great mistake to classify the *Atlas* solely as a document of Tibetan medicine. Instead, it stands as a general document of Tibetan culture, truly a unique encyclopedia of medieval Tibet that provides graphic descriptions of its culture and social structure and shares its wealth of knowledge regarding man and nature and the very phenomenon of life itself. The paintings are an invaluable key to the full legacy Tibet brings to the modern world, offering insights in a multitude of areas, including cultural studies, philosophy, theology, ethnography, history, medicine, pharmacology, botany, mineralogy, zoology, art history, music, and choreography.

The Tibetan view of the world is one of integration and unity. Tibetan medicine sees the physical and spiritual essence of man as a functionally integral structure that is also interconnected with nature, the cosmos, and society. Man is a part of nature, and for this reason he experiences the influence of all the forces of heaven and earth, the movements of the heavenly bodies and stars, the changing of the seasons, day and night, climate and landscape, mountains, waters, plants, and animals. He must correlate his way of life with the seasons of the year, the climate, and the demands of geography, wearing the right clothing, eating particular foods, balancing time spent in work and relaxation, and dwelling in the right home. The interaction between man and nature is limited by several taboos and moral prohibitions. One cannot dig the earth, break stones, chop down trees, foul water sources, or build dams without the permission of the spirits of the earth, trees, stones, and water, and this requires the appropriate rituals of sacrifice and penitential prayers. A bride's wedding procession, the erecting of houses and temples, the digging of graves and wells, and funeral procedures all require ritual permission and propitiation of the spirits of the earth. There is a belief that it is on the moral condition of people that the strength and weakness of their defenders depend, and one must have great regard for the deities of earth and heaven, mindful of the cataclysms of nature—floods, earthquakes, unseasonal storms, hail, downpours, hurricanes, deaths, fires, droughts, and so on.

The Four Tantras and the *Lapis Lazuli*

Working on such an extensive document of Tibetan culture, one so profound in content and so complex in form, one is impressed by the seamlessness of the whole: often the captions taken on their own are like mysterious cyphers, and can only be truly understood by reading the corresponding text in the *Four Tantras* and the *Lapis Lazuli.* Thus it seems worthwhile to review the nature of these texts, the fundamental doctrines of Tibetan medicine.

The *Atlas* follows their structure quite strictly. The first four paintings (1–4) explicate the content of the six chapters of the first volume of the *Lapis Lazuli;* the next thirty-three paintings (5–37) of the *Atlas* set forth the content of the thirty-one chapters of the second. The material of the ninety-two chapters of the third volume of the *Lapis Lazuli* is distributed among sixteen paintings (38–53) of the *Atlas.* The remaining twenty-four paintings (twenty-three in our set) cover the content of the fourth volume of the *Lapis Lazuli.*

The paintings in the *Atlas* are composed according to a precise scheme that is strictly maintained for all seventy-six paintings. In the top portion of each is its ordinal numeral and an indication as to which volume of the *Lapis Lazuli* the given painting pertains. Then follow the drawings, captions for them, and a summary of the painting's contents.

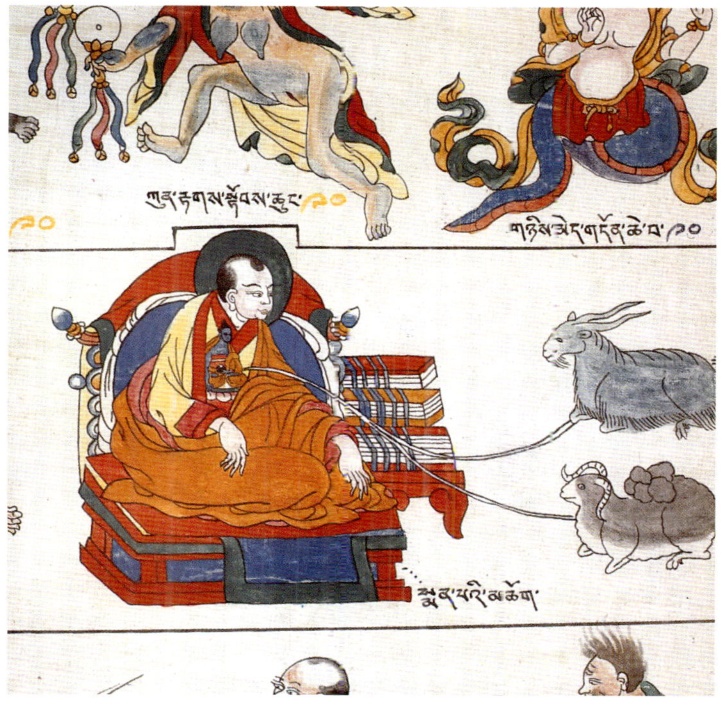

This illustration of the "topmost" physician shows him to be like the Buddha, who relieves all pain and diseases. Next to him may be seen the medical tantras, composed of leaves bundled in silk and tied (detail, pl. 40).

As has been detailed in Fernand Meyer's essay above, the theoretical and practical foundations of Tibetan medicine were originally set forth in a fundamental treatise entitled *The Four Tantras,* the full title of which is *The Eight Tantras of the Secret Oral Teachings, the Eight Branches, the Essence of the Elixir of Immortality.* Subsequently the *Four Tantras* received wide recognition and became the fundamental source text for Tibetan medicine, still used today.

In the full title of the *Four Tantras,* "eight branches" is a direct reference to the connection between the *Four Tantras* and the tradition of Indian Ayurvedic medicine, particularly the *Astangahrdaya Samhita,* the seventh-century text that was one of the basic sources used in compiling the *Four Tantras.* Characteristic of Indian medicine is the division of the entire body of medical texts into eight parts, or "branches": the structure of the body; conception, development of the fetus, and childhood diseases; female diseases; diseases caused by evil spirits; trauma; poisoning; old age; and the strengthening of male potency. It is interesting that the title itself contains no words indicating its relationship to medicine, a function evidently fulfilled by "eight branches," which served to define it as a medical treatise. Unlike the *Astangahrdaya Samhita,* the *Four Tantras*

This detail (pl. 35) shows the Instructional Tantra emanating from the Healing Buddha as the Buddha Ratnasambhava, whose mind represents the transformation of pride into "sameness."

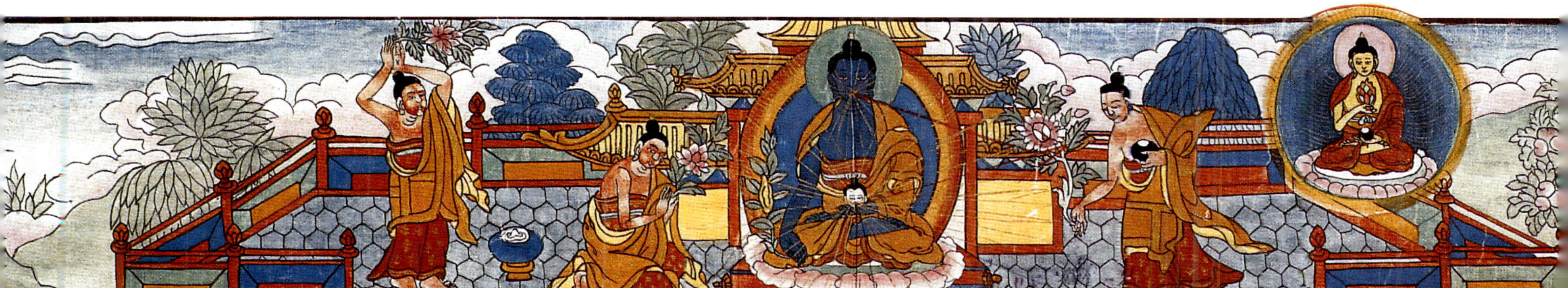

are divided into four major parts, here called *rgyud.* Let us consider this term, which was probably new to a medical text. The term owes its appearance to Tantrism, which by the time the *Four Tantras* were compiled by Yuthog Yontan Gonpo the Younger (1112–1203)—the twelfth century—had been the reigning form of Tibetan Buddhism for many centuries. It may be that the entire body of medical knowledge was divided into four parts, also called "tantras," by analogy with the division of the tantras in the Tibetan Buddhist canon: the Root Tantra *(rtsa rgyud),* the Explanatory Tantra *(shad-rgyud),* the Instructional Tantra *(man-ngag rgyud),* and the Subsequent Tantra *(phi ma-i rgyud).*

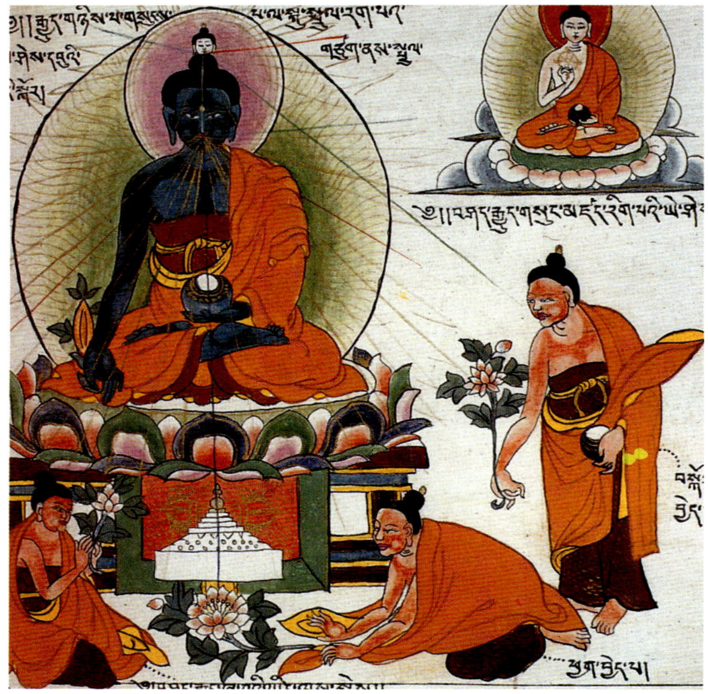

To deliver the second medical tantra, the Healing Buddha emanates multicolored rays of light that cleanse living beings of negativity and heal physical sufferings caused by humoral imbalance (detail, pl. 3).

The *Four Tantras* were set forth in the spirit of the teaching about *avataras,* who in this case represent the embodiment of various manifestations of a single individual. In order to tell the *Four Tantras,* Shakyamuni Buddha was reincarnated as Bhaisajyaguru, who emanated, in turn, five sages embodying his person in the essential aspects of body, speech, mind, actions, and qualities.

In the *Four Tantras,* especially the Explanatory Tantra, one encounters several attempts at a direct rethinking of the theoretical postulates of Ayurvedic medicine from the standpoint of the postulates of Tantrism. Like all tantric texts, the *Four Tantras* is protected from the uninitiated by the institution of initiation, the *dbang,* which by means of oaths and vows keeps information from leaking out of the circle of the elect. Because the word *rgyud* in the text's title is also the word for "tantra," we have translated the title as *The Four [Medical] Tantras.*

Among the retinue of the Medicine Buddha is the Hindu divinity Vajrapani, who embodies power (detail, pl. 1).

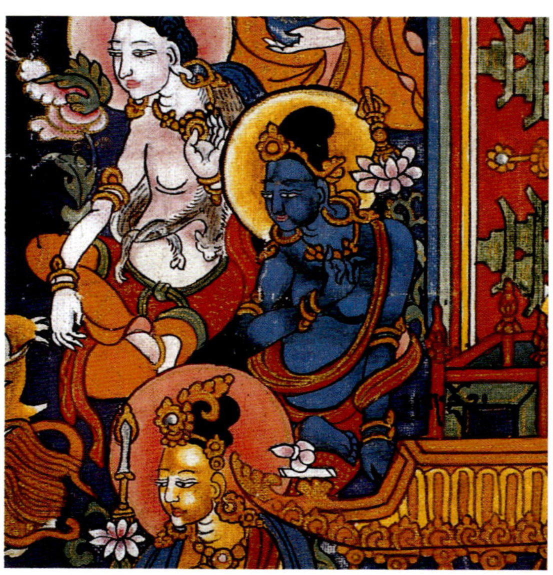

Tibetan historical literature provides no one opinion about the appearance of the *Four Tantras* in Tibet or its authorship. These issues are exceptionally important for our understanding of the specific nature of the theory and practice of Tibetan medicine, since all medical literature created after the *Four Tantras* was written as commentaries on them. There are two versions of the history of the *Four Tantras,* one mythological and one more or less historically accurate. According to the first version, the *Four Tantras* were set out by Shakyamuni Buddha during his four-year sojourn in a grove of medicinal plants located in the country of Oddiyana. Here Shakyamuni Buddha created the city of Sudarsana ("beautiful to behold") by his magic, building a palace out of five precious materials: gold, silver, white and red pearl, and vaidurya [beryl].[17]

In the center of the palace built of five precious materials, the Medicine Buddha, the Bhaisajyaguru, mounted the lapis lazuli throne surrounded by gods, sages, "outsiders" (non-Buddhists), and "insiders" (Buddhists), to whom he related all four parts of the *Four Tantras.* Each group understood in its own way, which is why there came to be four different traditions of medicine. The tradition of the gods was given the name the "Jug of Cure"; the tradition of the sages *(rishis),* the "Eight Divisions of Charaka"; the tradition of the non-Buddhists, the "Tantra of the Black Shiva"; and the tradition of the Buddhists, the "Division of the Three Protectors" (Mañjushri, Avalonikeshvara, and Vajrapani).

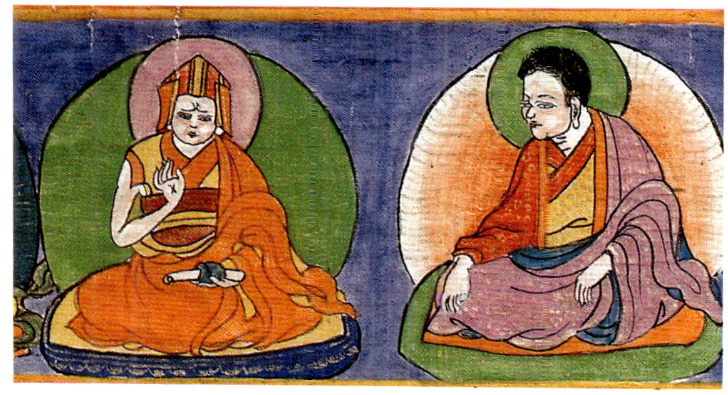

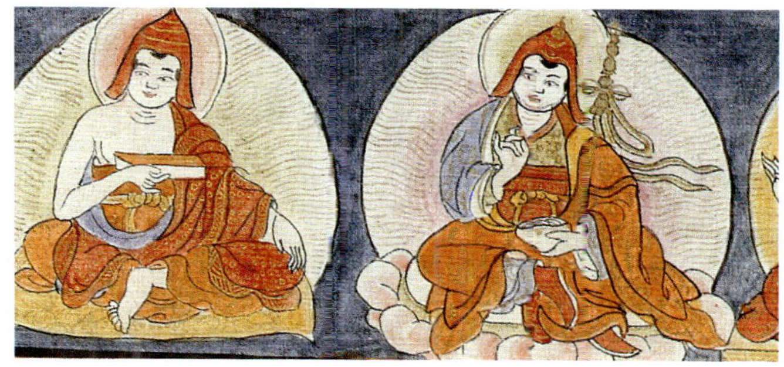

TOP: Chandrabhinandana, the great scholar of Kashmir (left), said to be one of the translators of the Four Tantras into Tibetan and Padmakara (detail, pl. 19). BOTTOM: King Trisong Detsen (left), who in the eighth century founded Melung, Country of Medicine, the first Tibetan medical college, and Mune, his son (detail, pl. 3).

Only *rishi* Rigpa'i-Ye-Shes—the personification of the speech of the Buddha—properly understood the teaching set forth by the Bhaisajyaguru, and the text he recorded was called the *Four Tantras,* which was destined to become the classical text of Tibetan medicine. It is said that it was written in lazulite ink on golden leaves and is kept to this day in Oddiyana. This was the original version of the text. There the Explanatory Tantra is recounted more or less in full. The Root Tantra was given in the form of an "enumeration," evidently, of the chapters of the entire treatise, and the third and fourth, the Instructional and Subsequent Tantras, were recounted only in part; practical medicine and pharmacology were left unfinished. Eventually this text reached the Kashmiri scholar Chandrabhinandana (eighth century), and the further dissemination of the *Four Tantras,* according to this legend, is linked with the names of various historical figures.

Tibetan medical sources say that in the eighth century a Tibetan translator, Vairocana, went to India, where together with Chandrabhinandana he translated the *Four Tantras* into Tibetan. The translation was carried to Tibet by Vairocana and presented as a gift to King Trisong Detsen (742–97), his son, and to Padmasambhava. During the construction of the first monastery in Tibet at Samye, the text was hidden in a vase-shaped column, where it was found 150 years later by a discoverer named Trapa Ngonshe. In time, the treatise was transmitted to Konchok Kyab, and later, passing from hand to hand, it reached Yuthog the Younger. From this we are to conclude that the text told by the Buddha Shakyamuni reached Yuthog the Younger in unaltered form.

The second version of the origin of the texts casts Yuthog the Younger as the author of the *Four Tantras.* It is thought that he creatively reworked texts in his possession that belonged to the Indian and Chinese medical traditions, creating an entirely new text entitled the *Four Tantras.* With time, the *Four Tantras* received high praise from Tibetan physicians and were recognized as the basic teaching tool for the training of traditional Tibetan doctors. Yuthog the Younger accomplished a titanic task. He made many additions to the Instructional Tantra and the Subsequent Tantra, included a chapter on medicines and a chapter on the physician in the Explanatory Tantra, and made several clarifications and changes.

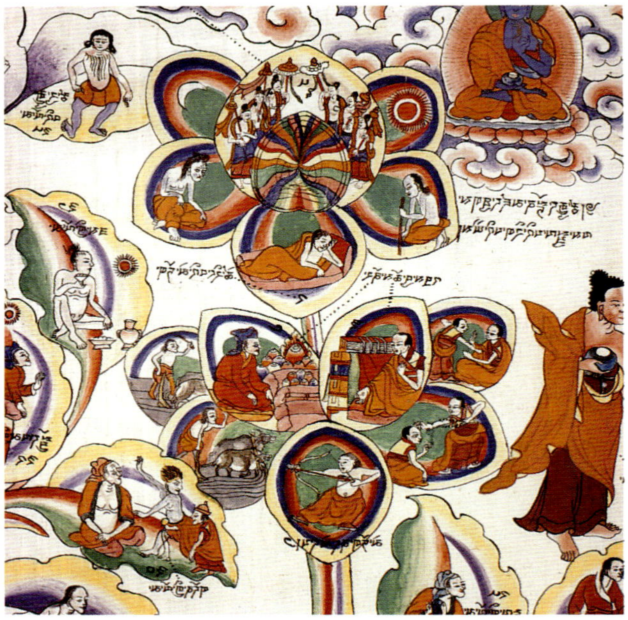

In this detail from plate 2, which illustrates chapter 2 of the Root Tantra, are seen flowers and fruit that symbolize freedom from disease, as well as spiritual well-being, longevity, enlightenment, and bliss.

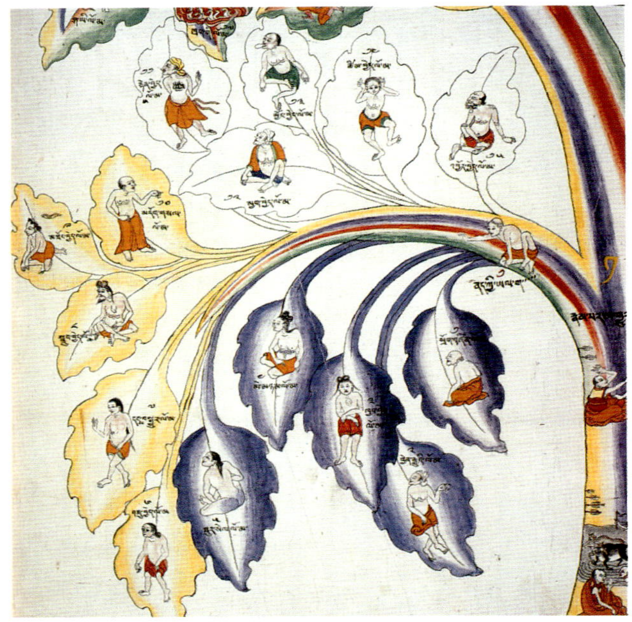

From this first branch of the Tree of Health and Disease (pl. 2) descend the leaves (right to left) of life-sustaining breath: ascending wind, pervasive wind, fire-accompanying wind, and descending purgative wind.

The Organization of the *Four Tantras*

The first volume of the *Four Tantras,* the Root Tantra, consists of six chapters, which set forth the legendary origin of medicine in Tibet, the causes of diseases, and the means of their treatment. It lists the titles in all four volumes and provides a description of the Tree of Health and Disease (previously referred to by John Avedon), which schematically correlates roots, trunk, branches, leaves, flowers, and fruits with the categories and concepts that make up the structure of Tibetan medicine.

The second volume, the Explanatory Tantra, contains thirty-one chapters outlining the theoretical issues of Tibetan medicine on the basis of an Indian medical tradition concerning the three "humors" or "elements" of the human body (*rlung, mkhris-pa,* and *bad-kan*), the signs of bodily deterioration, the causes of disease, and the conditions that give rise to diseases. These chapters describe the signs of and differences between diseases, as well as illustrating how best to live, giving recommendations on diet and methods of treatment. The last chapter of the second volume is devoted to describing the kind of person a physician should be.

The third volume, the Instructional Tantra, consists of fifteen practical sections in which there are a total of ninety-two chapters. Described are the humoral disorders of *rlung, mkhris-pa, bad-kan,* and their combinations, and diseases of the head, eyes, ears, nose, mouth, and goiter, as well as of the heart, lungs, liver, spleen, kidneys, stomach, and small and large intestines. Special sections focus on childhood and female diseases, the treatment of diseases caused by old age, and the strengthening of potency. Thus, the third volume of the *Four Tantras* provides a description of all the diseases known to Tibetan medical practitioners in the Middle Ages.

The fourth volume, the Subsequent Tantra, consists of twenty-seven chapters. Here the information scattered throughout the preceding volumes is systematized: diagnosis based on the investigation of the pulse and on urine examination; prescriptions; the preparation of medicines; indications for their application; and techniques for carrying out such treatment procedures as moxibustion, compresses, baths, embrocations, and acupuncture. Thus, the body of the *Four Tantras* consists of 154 chapters (including the conclusion and colophon, 156).

The Genius of Sangye Gyamtso, Regent of the Fifth Dalai Lama

As previously outlined by Fernand Meyer, the development of medicine in Tibet in the seventeenth century is linked with the name of the most prominent scholar of his day, Sangye Gyamtso (1653–1705), regent of the Fifth Dalai Lama (1617–82). In 1696, he founded the School of Medicine and Astrology on Chagpori Hill, which became one of the only educational institutions anywhere in Tibet where highly qualified traditional Tibetan physicians were trained within the framework of a united medical school. A special feature of this school was that Sangye Gyamtso worked out his own approach to Tibetan medicine as an integrated medical system, taking into consideration its unique structural, functional, and conceptual characteristics. He pioneered the new medical education in Tibet based on the study of the original written Tibetan medical sources and the commentary literature that over the course of many centuries had been created through the efforts of outstanding scholars and traditional physicians in medieval Tibet. The teachers at Chagpori were monks sent there from other monasteries in Tibet. In addition to the purely medical disciplines, liturgy and spiritual practice occupied an important place.

As a prominent political figure and a great Buddhist scholar—an encyclopedist of medieval Tibet—Sangye Gyamtso applied great efforts to rallying the Tibetan clergy. With this goal in mind, and being a theologian, he tackled the unification of the teachings of the various then-extant schools on the subjects within his scholarly competence. In 1685, he completed a text on astrology begun two years before, the *White Beryl,* which chronicles the principal events in the history of Buddhism. In 1698, he wrote the *Yellow Beryl,* in which the country's history is set forth as the history of the leading Gelugpa order.[18] In 1687, Gyamtso began writing the *Vaidur'ya yasel,* in which the author formulated his responses to the objections made by opponents after the publication of his *White Beryl.*

Of greatest interest to us are the medical works of Sangye Gyamtso: his practical oversight of the *Lhantab,* written in 1690 as a supplement to the third volume of the *Four Tantras* to address all the disputed issues of practical Tibetan medicine; the *Khogbug* (1702), on the history of medicine; the *Atlas of Tibetan Medicine;* and the most complete commentary on the *Four Tantras*—the *Lapis Lazuli,* written between

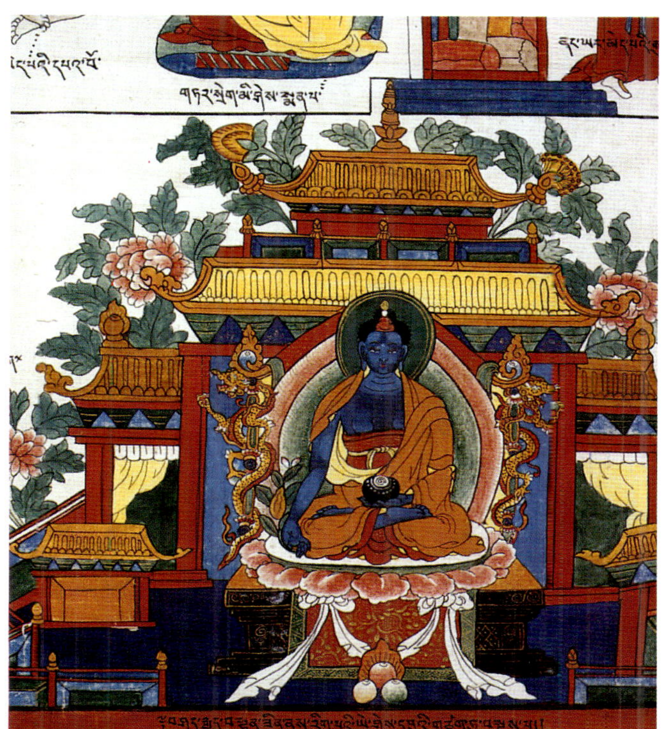

This detail concludes the painting that illustrates the good physician (pl. 40), who achieves happiness in this life. This image shows how, at the close of the Explanatory Tantra, the teaching is absorbed back into the crown of the Healing Buddha.

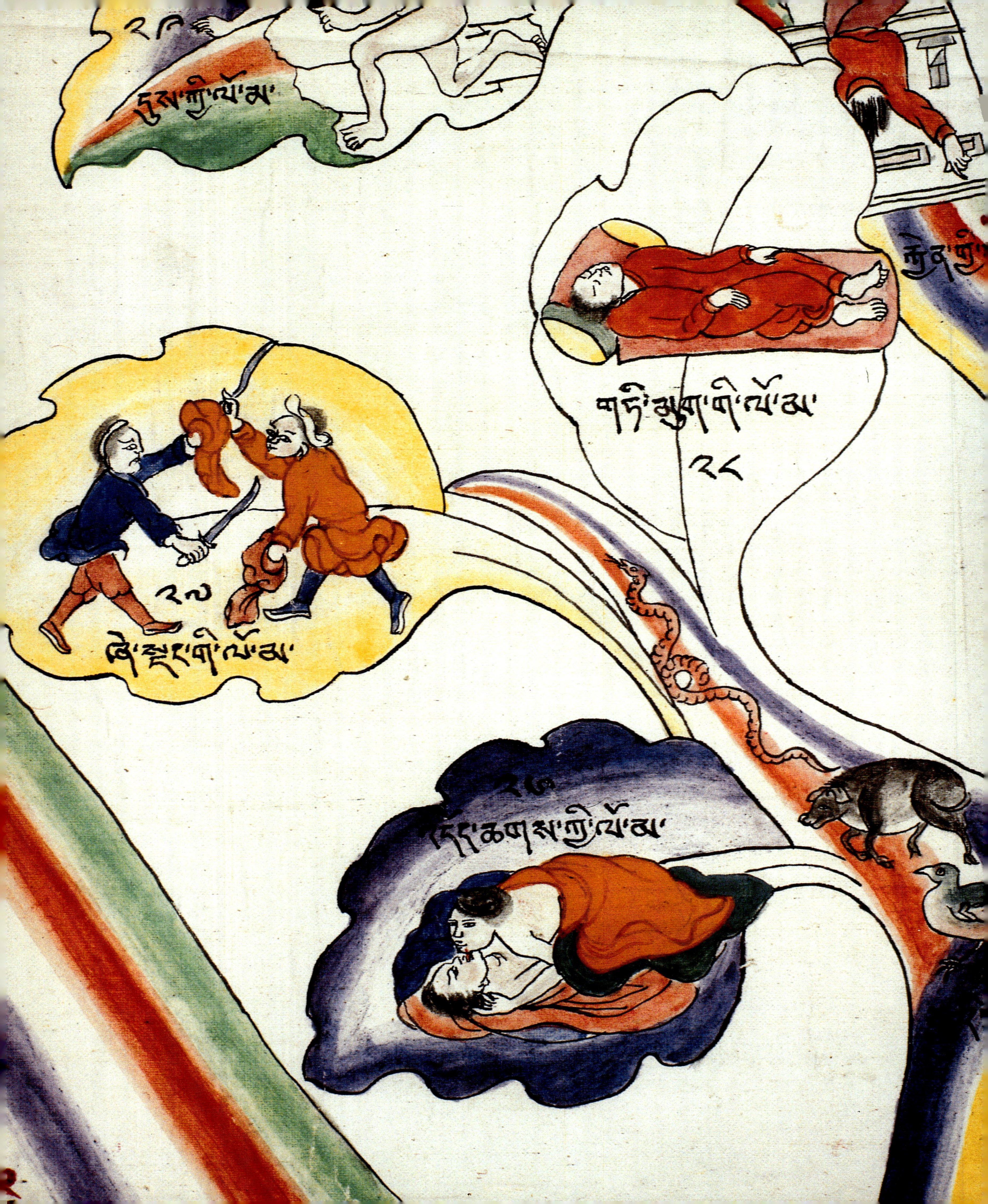

༢༩
དུས་ཀྱི་ལོ་མ་
ཀྱེན་ཀྱི
གཉི་ལུག་གི་ལོ་མ་
༢༨
༢༧
ཞེ་སྡང་གི་ལོ་མ་
༢༦
ད་ཆགས་ཀྱི་ལོ་མ་

1687 and 1688 and consisting of 4 volumes and 156 chapters, with each structural unit of the text serving as commentary on the corresponding section of the *Four Tantras.* The *Lapis Lazuli* was based on a large number of sources belonging to the ancient Indian, Chinese, and Tibetan medical traditions. In this work, Sangye Gyamtso showed himself to be the most important thinker in medieval Tibet, a subtle connoisseur of the theory and practice of Tibetan medical science.[19]

Subsequently, the *Lapis Lazuli* was recognized as a canonical treatise and included in the body of the second part of the Tibetan Buddhist canon, the *Tangyur* of Derge, which was published in the first half of the eighteenth century in eastern Tibet, in the principality of Derge.[20]

While the *Four Tantras* presents the traditions of Indian medicine, the *Lapis Lazuli* draws upon the experience of various oriental medical systems, in particular, the Indian and Chinese traditions. These are not only synthesized and reworked but are also coordinated with the way of life of the Tibetan people, their outlooks, customs, beliefs, and rituals. The *Lapis Lazuli* defines the specific ways in which the issues of health, disease, life, and death were posed and treated in Tibetan medicine in the seventeenth and eighteenth centuries.

Simultaneously with the writing of the *Lapis Lazuli* as an extensive commentary on the *Four Tantras,* the *Atlas of Tibetan Medicine* was created as an essential addition to the anatomical paintings and classification schemes traditionally used as teaching tools in monastic medical schools. Both the colophon of the *Lapis Lazuli* and the text of the *Khogbug* provide information on the elaboration and compilation of this set of visual aids on Tibetan medicine, which unlike previous instructional paintings were meant to serve as a graphic commentary on the subject matter of the volumes of the *Four Tantras.* Regarding the artists who realized Gyamtso's vision, the colophon of the *Lapis Lazuli* indicates that sixty of the paintings were executed by the graphic artist and printer Tendzin Norbuchen, "the reincarnate master of Lho-brag," and the painter Genyen of Lhasa (the former also created the graphic illustrations for the *White Beryl*). The Tibetan edition of the *Atlas of Tibetan Medicine* furthers the identification: Sangye Gyamtso is called the creator of the original *Atlas,* Tendzin Norbuchen of Lho-brag the graphic illustrator, and Genyen of Lhasa the colorist.[21] The seventy-nine paintings mentioned in the *Khogbug* actually illustrate the content of the *Blue Beryl,* that is, not only the subject matter of the *Four Tantras* but also what was in Sangye Gyamtso's commentary. In the final edition Shonnu Chakpa Chophel took an active part, adding quotations from and references to canonical literature and linking the tenets of medicine to the dogmas of tantric teaching.

The *Atlas of Tibetan Medicine* is an extraordinary work, bearing the stamp of a gifted and spiritually multifaceted author. In its functions both as a teaching and as an illustrative commentary to the *Four Tantras,* it makes myriad connections between medicine, culture, and the society of that era. It is these features that set the *Atlas* apart from other medical visual aids that existed before its appearance. The creation of the *Atlas* began in 1687 and was completed in 1688, when Sangye Gyamtso was either thirty-five or thirty-six years old. Various stages in this work are connected with the names of Gonchog Choidag, Panchen Lama of the Namgyal Monastery, and Shonnu Chakpa Chophel. In our opinion, it seems probable that Sangye Gyamtso conceived of creating a medical commentary in drawings from what he learned during the time when he was called Apti, a name that may be connected with some special instruction he received. According to custom, initiation into new cults and new spheres of knowledge entailed the receiving of a new name; thus one can to some extent gauge the interests and scholarly achievements of a

The three poisons of desire, hatred, and delusion, the primary causes of disease. On the right they are symbolically depicted as a bird, a snake, and a pig, respectively (detail, pl. 2).

Plant and animal materia medica; animal products are used very rarely in Tibetan medicine. The top register from left to right features four-o-clock root, rennet, and Solomon's seal (detail, pl. 27).

given individual by how many new names he has received. Among the gallery of deities and historical figures depicted in the first fifteen paintings of the *Atlas,* we find depictions of Apti[22] (Sangye Gyamtso) and Shonnu Chakpa Chophel (not pictured in this volume). This line of succession of medical knowledge goes back to the Fifth Dalai Lama. The caption under the depiction of Apti reads: "Apti, who unerringly transposed the content of the *Four Tantras,* putting a child's trust in the sages of this country." In the *Lapis Lazuli,* Sangye Gyamtso calls himself "Buddha Apti." The colophons to the *White Beryl* and the *Khogbug* also indicate that in Sanskrit his name was Buddha Apti, whereas in the Land of Snows it was Sangye Gyamtso. The *Khogbug* informs us that the name "Sangye Gyamtso" indicates his knowledge of the science of *vyakarana.* The structure of the name that refers to this period in Sangye Gyamtso's biography underscores his youth, his young mind's tendency toward the poetic, and his youthful self-confidence. In the *Khogbug,* Gyamtso writes that by the age of thirty-four he had studied ten sciences[23] and demonstrated special interest in everything that had to do with the science and art of the word (grammar, vocabulary, the study of synonyms, semantics, metrics, the theory of poetry), the art of painting and sculpture, medicine, and astrology. Ever since he was a child he had been interested in plants, studying and drawing them. He was thus the ideal person to present such an integrated view of Tibetan culture.

Medicine as an Integrated Discipline

In the *Atlas of Tibetan Medicine,* autonomous drawings are united by the logic of the medical context.[24] K. M. Gerasimova was the first scholar in the field of Tibetan studies to examine the iconography in the *Atlas* as an aesthetic teaching about the regularities of the proportional structure of the body. She also realized that the *Atlas* may be regarded as a general reference on Tibetan ethnography, characterizing it as a historical document in the integral context of medieval Tibetan culture.

In 1968, source and field research on the theory and practice of Tibetan medicine began in Ulan-Ude, study that is now concentrated at the Institute of Biology at the Buryat Scientific Center (part of the Siberian Division of the Russian Academy of Sciences in Ulan-Ude). The division's principal aims are to acquire new medicinal preparations, clarify methodological approaches in drug therapy for disease, and utilize the *Atlas's* valuable recommendations for the preservation and strengthening of human health. The success of the medical-biological research has been facilitated by the scientific translation and intensive study of Tibetan medical texts, as well as by orientalist and anthropological research. Historical analysis is vital for assessing the very complex world view represented in these paintings; it is necessary for a real understanding of both the theory and the practice of Tibetan medicine. It is also essential for contemplating the unique mix of the rational and irrational in traditional medicine.

Analysis of the *Atlas* as a historical document of Tibetan culture reveals a remarkable vision of man as a biological and social being, regarded from many points of view and in the context of the actual ways of life that once existed in Tibet. The value of these paintings is thus not confined to the theory and practice of medicine, teachings about health and the causes of illness, or medical treatments for various ailments. All of this medical knowledge is based on profound ideas regarding the nature of life itself, both physical and spiritual aspects; what

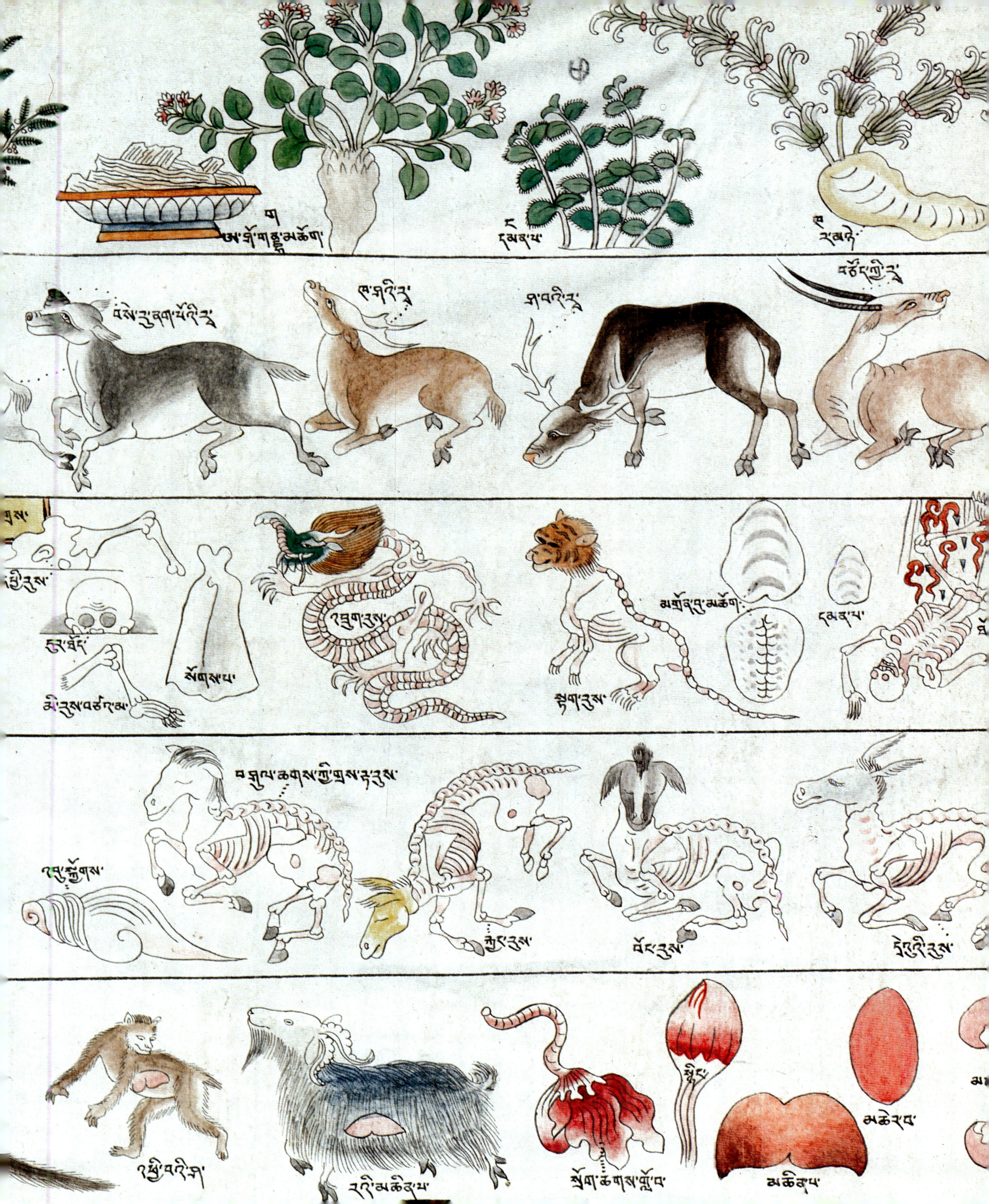

ཀ
ང
དམན་པ།
ཁ
ར་མཉེ
བསེ་རུ་ནག་པོའི་རྭ།
ཤ་བའི་རྭ།
ཧར་སྦོང་།
སོགས་པ།
འབྲུག་རུས།
སྟག་རུས།
དམན་པ།
རྐྱང་རུས།
བོང་རུས།
དྲེའུའི་རུས།
ར་འི་མཆིན་པ།
མཆེར་པ།
མཆིན་པ།

precisely makes a human being vital, active, and capable of growth and reproduction; why man dies; and what happens to the body and soul after death.

As we have discussed, the *Four Tantras,* the *Lapis Lazuli,* and the *Atlas of Tibetan Medicine* represent a synthesis of classical Indian and Chinese medical knowledge reworked in accordance with Tibetan Buddhism and taking into consideration Tibet's popular customs, beliefs, and general outlooks. At the same time, the *Atlas* documents the general level of development of the natural sciences and the philosophical world view of seventeenth- and eighteenth-century Tibetan society. Sangye Gyamtso examines the science of medicine within the system of the eighteen sciences of the ancient and medieval culture of India and Tibet. He cites two sets of eighteen sciences in the tradition of the *Vinayavasta Sutra* referring to the period of the first prophecy of Shakyamuni Buddha, and of the *Abhidharmakosha* in the fifth century.

The enumeration of the Vinaya sciences includes various philosophical and religious teachings from Indian antiquity: the Vedas, tantra, yoga, linguistic and philological sciences, logic, dialectics, astrology, the theory of ceremonial ritual, and so on.

The classification of the sciences of the *Abhidharmakosha* focuses on such scientific disciplines as arithmetic, mathematics, astronomy, calendrical and astrological calculations, linguistics, poetry, art, music, medicine, logic, and dialectics, but here we also have the techniques of archery, the rules of ritual and sacrifice, and the lore of wizardry and sexual life. The eighteenth-century Tibetan classification of sciences is called *"The Eighteen Spheres of Knowledge of the Inner and Outer World of Man."* This elegant system includes technology, or the knowledge of the general laws of construction of the world; the sciences of the universe and the six forms of animate beings; the laws of appearance; the laws of time, or the knowledge of past, present, and future life; the laws of death, or the continuity of rebirths conditioned by the sinfulness of beings; moral norms; the science of consciousness, or the knowledge of the three degrees of intellect (higher, middle, and lower); the sciences of perception and spiritual improvement; dogma; the knowledge of the *bodhi* as the instantaneous departure from *samsara* (the cycle of rebirth); and the means of universal purification and sanctification. Cited are such sciences as medicine, pharmacology, grammar, and dialectics. Sangye Gyamtso thus reviews the full system of basic views of the world that were fundamental for every Buddhist in Tibet.

Divine Proportion

This indissoluble link between medicine and the overall level of spiritual development in India and among the peoples of central Asia can be divined in many of the visual characteristics of the *Atlas of Tibetan Medicine.* In particular, one can point to the interrelationship between the medical, anthropological, and aesthetic sciences. In India, ancient physicians elaborated anthropometric systems for the various physical types. This knowledge lay at the base of iconometry—the canon of proportions used in the creation of art. Indian and Tibetan iconographic treatises appeared as a result of a centuries-long elaboration of the theory of Buddhist art, the main content of which is defined by the philosophical-aesthetic category of measure (see plate 4). The theory of measure—the teaching concerning the essential signs *(mtshan nyid)* of the qualitative and quantitative definition of objects and phenomenon—influenced the construction of the human figure in art.

The "measure of man" on the whole follows the Indian tradition of the iconographic modeling of the perfection of the gods' physical and spiritual beauty, while taking into consideration changes in the rules of Tibetan iconography. In the *Atlas,* the diagrams of human anatomy and physiology ordinarily depict man standing upright with his arms stretched out to the sides. This is the formula of N'yagrodhi, the Tree of N'yagrodha, the height of whose trunk is equal to the breadth of its crown, symbolizing the principle of perfect physical proportions, where the height of the body equals the span of the arms.

Unlike the higher category of gods, whose bodily proportions are calculated according to the system of ten palms (the palm being the unit of measurement), man is shorter and constructed disproportionately—the height of his body is less than the span of his arms. Only the *chakravartin,* the ideal man, the equal of the gods, can be as beautifully proportioned as a god, albeit based on a scale of only nine palms.

This medical systematization relies upon the basic premise of the scientific understanding of the world: the desire to count, measure, and group everything according to types, to break a whole down into its component parts, to combine the similar and separate the dissimilar. Fernand Meyer, in his introductory essay to the paintings, traces the basic contours of this system of humors *(nyes-pas)* and powers. Additionally, we note that the *Atlas* classifies people by age, sex, state of health, external appearance, character, temperament, state of moral consciousness, and behavior. The distinguishing of people by appearance, temperament, spiritual capacities, morals, conduct, longevity, and the nature of their worldly destiny is defined in terms of their deviations from the normal, or ideal, combination of the humors within the human being.

This detail from the Tree of Health and Disease (pl. 2) illustrates the three humors (wind, bile, and phlegm), as well as adipose, bone, and marrow tissue, the reproductive fluids, and excretion.

In its ideas about man's physical and spiritual constitution, ancient ontological traditions are interwoven with later medieval traditions. The Ayurvedic formula of the "three foundations of life" took shape in antiquity: "One is in the head and the whole body; another is the breath and its support; and still another roams like *bla.*" The first two sites speak to the physical foundation of the vitality of the human organism; the third refers to the soul, the animistic foundation of life. The traditional notion of the supernatural vital qualities of the body and head comes out in the extensive ethnographic material on burial and memorial rituals and customs of embalming, mummification, protective face coverings, and clay, silver, and gold masks, inasmuch as the head was ascribed the magical power of vitality and life-giving potential.

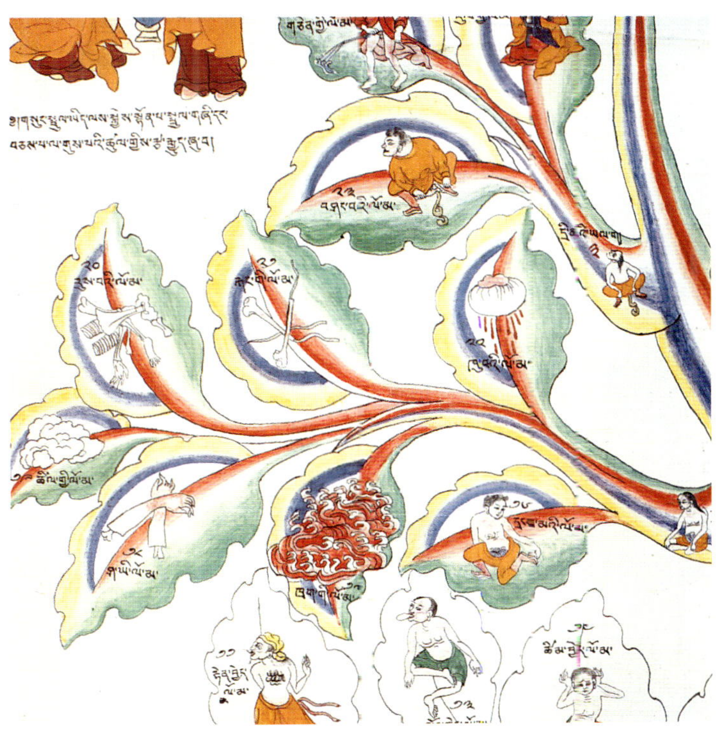

A Comparison of the Ayurvedic and Tibetan Traditions

Sangye Gyamtso comments on the Ayurvedic tradition, citing the *Kalachakra Tantra* and its basic commentary, the *Dri-med.* He does not explain the meaning of Ayurveda or the three

The heart chakra (dharmachakra), through which the consciousness of the senses flows (detail, pl. 7).

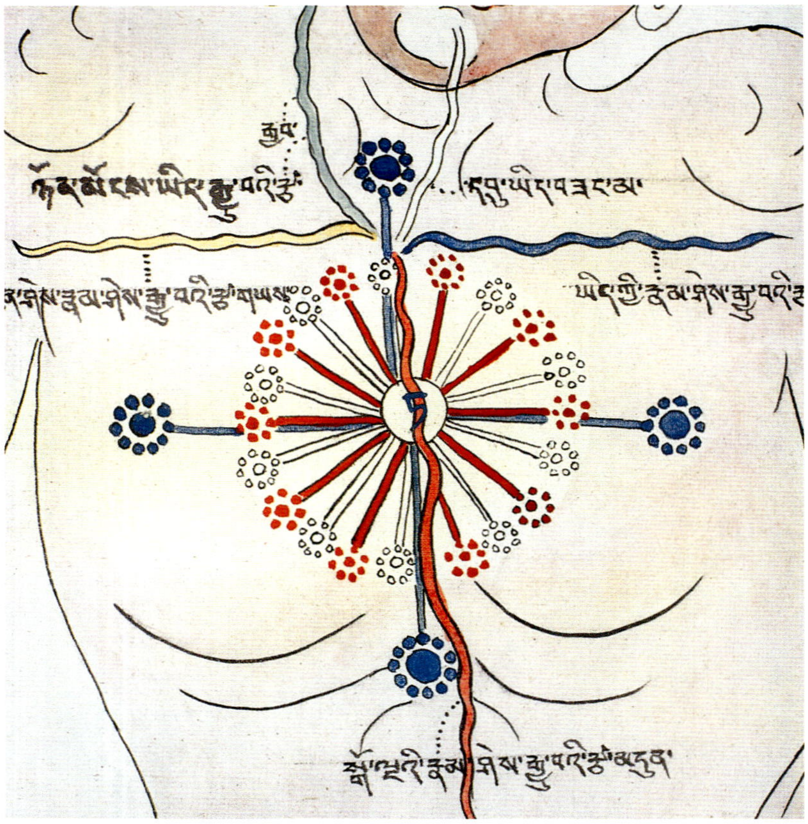

foundations of life, but interprets these from a contemporary tantric medical perspective, reducing the Ayurvedic formula to the question of a life-essence or lifespan principle that circulates in the body.

Alluding to the commentaries of the *Kalachakra Tantra,* the *Lapis Lazuli* states that in the vessels there circulates the "essence" of digested food, which is transformed into sperm. On its way through the chakras (points at which the channels intertwine; see plates 9 and 10), the sperm is concentrated into a mystical fluid called *byan chub sems-kyi khams.* According to the tradition of the medical treatise *(sMan dbyang-lugs),* this particular substantiation is called *bla,* which also circulates, changing place in the body daily and in the course of a lunar month completing a full rotation from the toe of the left foot in men (the right in women) to the toe of the right foot (left in women). In the *Lapis Lazuli,* however, the description of this cycle of transpositions of *bla* involves the articulations of the skeleton rather than the vessels. Here the Ayurvedic and the Tibetan traditions of designating the sites of substance circulation conflict: according to one, it is a matter of vessels; according to the other, bones.

In Indian Vedic language, there is a term *prana,* which signifies the life force of man and refers to the five types of breath, the sensory organs and their functions, and the structure of the human organism. The seven *pranas* are the two eyes, two ears, two nostrils, and mouth. Life forces are known both as *pranas* and as *atmans.* The *Taittiriya-Upanishad* sets forth a thesis on the hierarchy and totality of individual inner *atmans* of the physical and spiritual constitution of man: the *atman* consisting of the juices of food, the *atman* consisting of the breath, the *atman* consisting of reason, and the *atman* of discernment and bliss. The breath as the life force, on the one hand, is identified with the force of the intellect; the knowing *atman,* on the other, is looked upon as a factor in the physiological activity of the organs. As a vital principle, the breath is connected with the *atman* in the heart and with the system of vessels through which the breath moves throughout the body.

In Tibetan medical sources we recognize all these ancient Indian ideas, though in a form influenced by Chinese medical theories. Tibetan treatises talk not about *prana* but about various types of *rlung,* which are not identical with the *rlung* humor. The five kinds of *rlung* provide for speech, the motor functions of the muscles, digestion, and the disposal of the excretions of the sexual and digestive organs. The first and most important type is *srog-'dzin,* "the holder, the bearer of life," based in the heart and providing for the breath and for clarity of the sensory and ra-

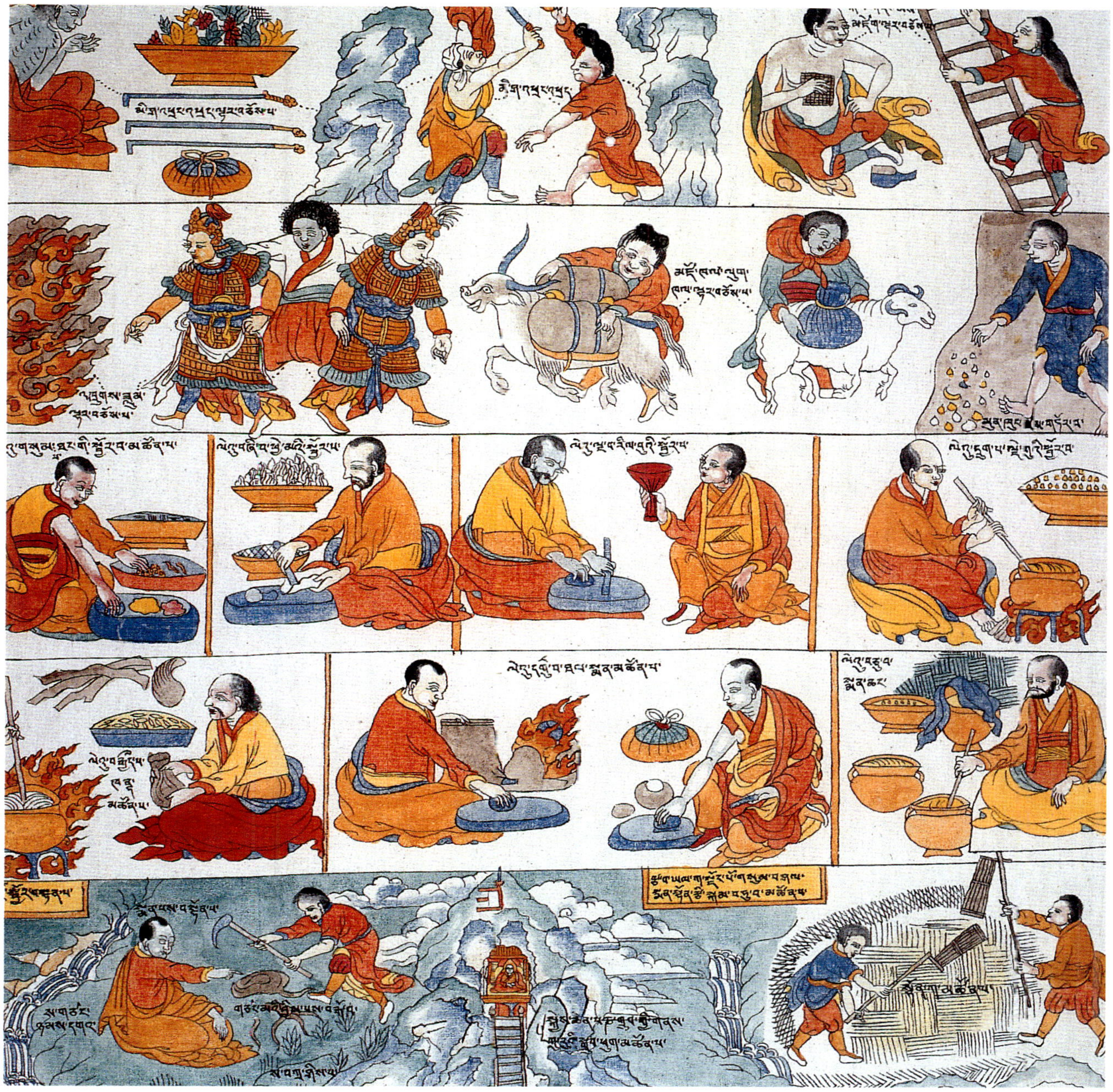

In the lower register of this detail (pl. 28) are seen the sort of places where medicines may be found: a clean and pleasant, auspicious ground where scholars and masters gather. A "pure child" digs up the herbs.

tional activities of consciousness. *Rlung* is divided into the crude material type (functional, operational *rlung*) and the "*rlung* of consciousness," the extremely subtle spiritual substantiation that forms an absolute concentration of life force in the heart, or an essence of absolute life potential, which is transported by the substantiation of the energy of *rlung*. Readers of the *Tibetan Book of the Dead (Bardo thödol)* will recognize this "essence of life" as that which leaves the *avadhuti* through the *Brahma* opening in the skull after death and lands in the beyond-the-grave world of the *bardo*, where after several transformations in the course of forty-nine days it is reborn to new life, grapples with the father's sperm and the mother's blood, and acquires corporeal flesh during the development of the fetus in the mother's womb.

In plate 6 (and in painting 12; unillustrated), a substance indicated by the letter *a* circulates in the vessels of the heart system. This is the blood. The pulsing vessels at the base of the throat,

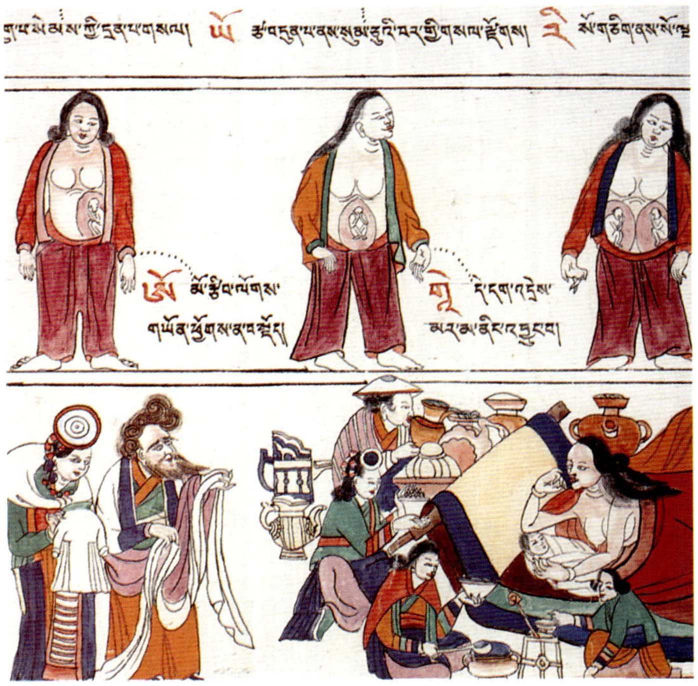

Above: In the upper images are seen the positions of the male, female, and hermaphrodite; below, the proper care of the mother after delivery of the baby is seen. A woman who has known childbirth cuts the cord, and the right foods are brought to the new mother (detail, pl. 3).

Below: This detail from the "Conduct" painting (pl. 21) includes illustrations of the wrong sort of behavior: sitting on the scriptures, destroying sacred images, committing murder and theft, and engaging in sexual intercourse in broad daylight, or with a woman who is not one's wife.

wrist, and middle finger are designated as the "*bla* vessels." In the unillustrated painting, the pulsing vessel from the wrist to the end of the middle finger is joined by a dotted line to the caption of the third thesis of Ayurveda: "According to the tradition of the tantras and the Ayurveda, the basis of life is *bla,* wandering." It is no accident that the inscription is placed here. The *Lapis Lazuli* indicates that *bla* emerges from the vessel of the middle finger at night during sleep or illness and can be caught by an evil spirit, which is why people wear bracelets and rings as amulets.

From the material in the *Atlas* and the *Lapis Lazuli,* we discover a similarity between the terms *a, bla,* and *mdangs,* that is, that which circulates in the vessels and bones of the human body. When all the juices of the seven bodily constitutents become sperm and menstrual blood, the total life force arises—*mdangs,* "the shining of life and health." Based in the middle of the heart, *mdangs* fills the body with vital energy and can also "wander"—detach from the body during sleep and be caught by an evil spirit.

The terms cited above signify not simply blood or some bodily life force but that which is approximately called the "soul." The term *a* in the *Lapis Lazuli* appears in the combination *a-thung* (short *a*), meaning both "menstrual blood" and the spirit that quits the body during death. In the funeral ritual it is returned to the deceased through the skull to the heart, thereby reanimating the dead person to "listen" to the lama's after-death teaching.

The similarity of these concepts from various traditions attests not only to the combining of ideas from different periods but also to a commonality in the paramount spiritual ground they share. In all, the physical body retreats into the background: man's physical being can be alive only given animation. The *Atlas* and Tibetan medical treatises in general demonstrate the development

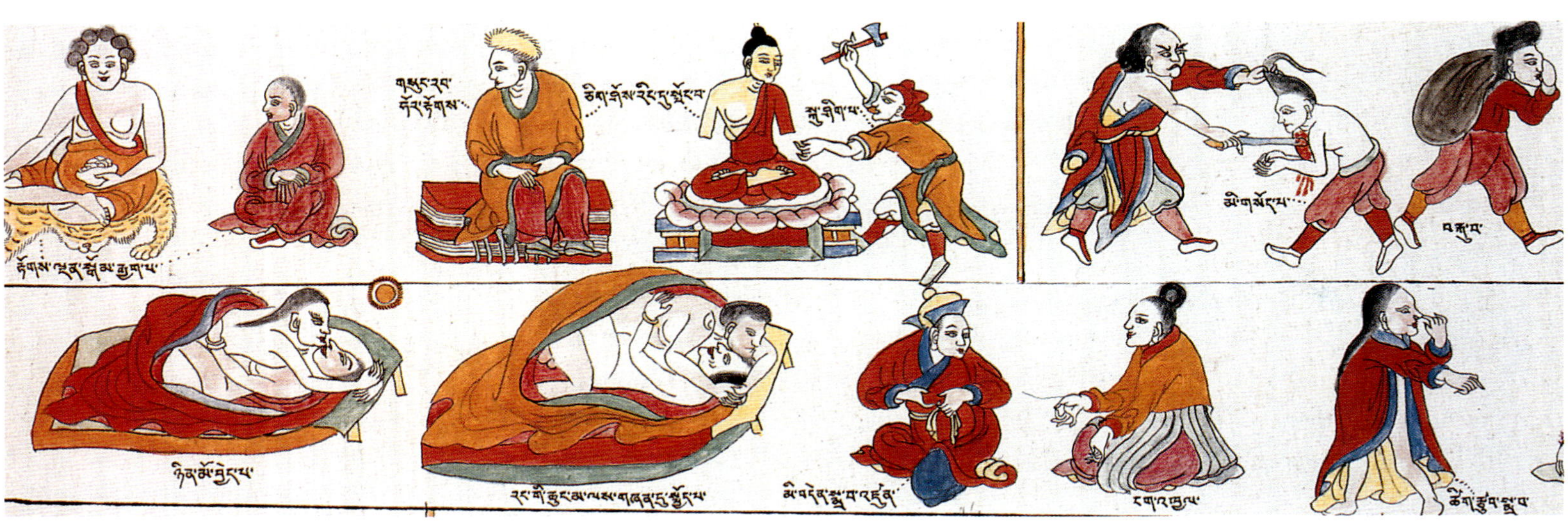

of ideas about the spiritual factor of vitality. The doctrinal rejection in early Buddhism of the existence of an immortal and immutable soul in man was replaced by heightened attention to the forms and functions of consciousness. The consciousness that is created through sensory perception is considered the lowest form of consciousness, inseparable from bodily functions. It cannot be "reborn" from one life to another or be free in the living and dying man. It is the "rational consciousness" that possesses these qualities, functioning during sleep and death and in the beyond-the-grave world of the *bardo.*

A characterization of the various types of consciousness, including the sensual, can be found in the *Atlas* in plates 7, 14, and 39, which give information about the *chakra* of the heart, dreams, and psychological illnesses. Plate 14 depicts the points where the soul leaves the body during dreaming sleep: through the sinciput and the eyes, in four directions from the heart, and through the anus in three downward directions. The soul visits different worlds depending on which point of the body it leaves through during sleep, and it sees corresponding dreams about the worlds of gods, people, animals, the beyond-the-grave world, hell, and the sphere of *preta.* Through these points, the soul can leave the body during death as well.

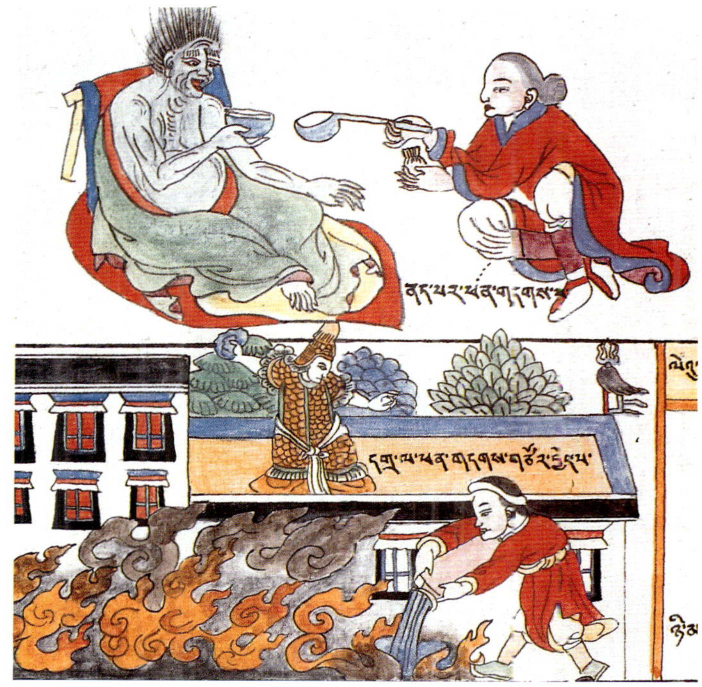

Good conduct demands that one assist invalids and "emphatically" assist one's own enemies (detail, pl. 21).

In the medical texts, death is described as the process of deterioration of the primary elements, the gradual extinguishing of the activity of the sensory organs, the transformation and concentration in the heart of all the vital "winds" into an indivisible, integral "essence of life" that quits the deceased, ideally, through the *avadhuti* and the Brahma opening. The process of death and the return to life are analogous, but occur in reverse order. The neverending circle of life and death in *samsara* can be broken by a radical cleansing of karma or special tantric rituals.

Judging from the *Four Tantras,* half of the illnesses known to the Tibetans were attributed to the effect of harmful deities and spirits, as karmic punishment for violating various taboos and rules of religious morality. Traditional beliefs and outlooks not only retained their force in popular customs but also entered the system of Tibetan medicine. Since antiquity, the practice of divination and prediction had played a major role in the treatment of diseases, the elimination of various misfortunes and unfavorable circumstances, and the prognosis of success or failure in everyday matters. For the medieval doctor, divination was one method of diagnosis, a way to determine the causes of an illness. It was important to establish precisely which demonic forces were harming the patient's health in order to eliminate their injurious influence by means of rituals of propitiation, elimination, and suppression. In the *Atlas* there are many classifications of harmful supernatural forces: fifteen devils causing childhood illnesses; eighteen types of spirits of the deceased; eight types of gods and spirits of the traditional religions of India and Tibet; 3,601,080 evil spirits inflicting harm on nature and people; and so on. A diagnosis of the causes and nature of illnesses by means of divination from urine poured into a cup brings out the effect of evil spirits in the social sphere (see plate 17). Here is where the deities and spirits of the people's pre-Buddhist beliefs operate. The protective recommendations of physicians consist of designating various religious rituals. The *Atlas* shows rituals for protecting life that

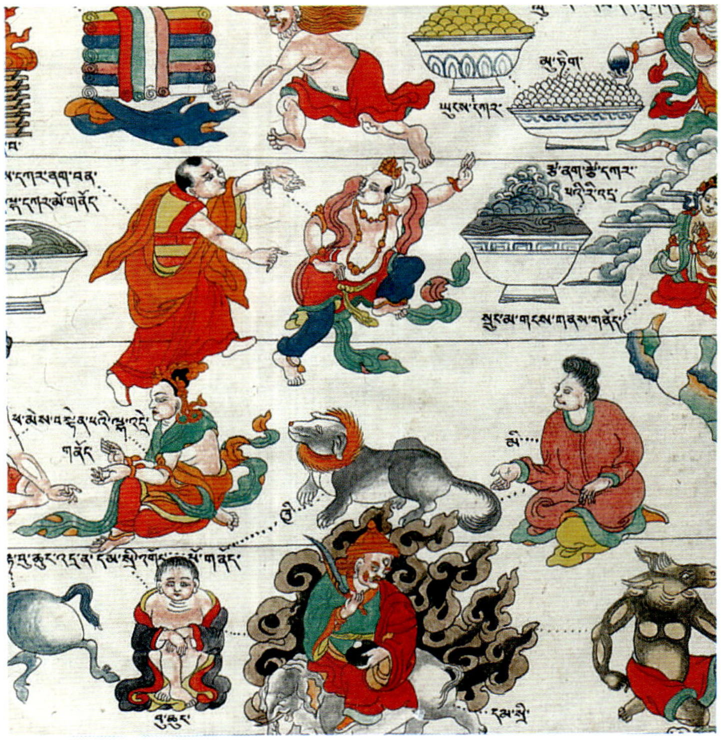

The ancient divining science finds in the reading of urine vapor the White Goddess known both to Buddhists and practitioners of Bön, as well as gods and demons served by one's paternal ancestors (detail, pl. 17).

are derived from various religious practices, including Bön, Buddhist Indian cults, Tibetan black-hat, red-hat, and yellow-hat sects, and tantric sorcerers—the so-called *sangasva*—who swear death-dealing oaths and perform rituals to suppress the demons of earth and water.

The Art of the *Atlas*

Canonical cult art has strict rules for the frontal construction of the figure of a deity. This may be seen in the impassive images of buddhas and boddhisatvas, as well as in the static expressions of the gods who defend the Buddhist religion and its followers. Given this reality, the drawings of the *Atlas* are truly exceptional; they present a rare set of secular subjects whose artistic resolution is free of the standard clichés for the depiction of sacred objects. Man is shown in the multiplicity of his everyday situations, in the freedom of his body's range of movement. At the same time, it is essential to point out the influence of the general level of Buddhist artistic culture, the achievements in the sphere of anatomical accuracy in the depictions of the human body, the idealization of the image, and the understanding of compositional means of expression, dynamics, and decoration. What makes the graphic texture of the *Atlas* unique is the fragmentation and autonomy of its topics and drawings, inasmuch as they are unified not by thematic composition but by the "outside-the-frame" logic of a consecutive illustrative explication of the content of a medical treatise, a "translation" of a written text into the language of graphic signs. This informational substitution for the subject, action, and phenomenon by a specific manner, model, and sign fulfills the task of fixing and conveying knowledge and elaborating a widely accessible methodology for the teaching and practical utilization of the treatise by ordinary physicians without them having to delve into the sphere of philology and philosophy.

The sign system of the *Atlas* involves various levels of formalization of the language of substantive information by means of iconographic, schematic, and conventional signs. The iconographic signs convey the graphically real image; for example, seasonal phenomena in nature and human economic activity. Often, however, the realistic image has a conventional rather than a literal meaning. For example, drawings realistically depicting the earth being dug up, trees being chopped down, stones being broken up, and water sources being fouled point to the supernatural causes of diseases brought down by the anger of the "offended" spirits of the earth, water, trees, and stones. Other examples of the shift of iconographic signs into the rank of conventional and symbolic signs involve models: the sun's disc in an aureole of light means "day" and "noon" but also "good," "fine," "favorable." The signs for "mountain," "tree," "fortress," and "weapon" divined during the process of divination from urine indicate the influence of ancestral spirits. The staff used to summon the spirits of the ancestors, with ribbons at its upper end, indicates a prognosis: "what is desired will happen" or "what is desired will not happen." If the *badan* is in a vertical position with streaming ribbons, it means that the ancestors have heard the prayer and will help; a horizontal position for the staff with furled ribbons says that the gods did not hear the prayer, therefore "what is desired will not happen." The content of conventional signs is conditioned either by the realities of religious ideas and cult practice or else by images of mythology. Without taking the traditional mentality into consideration or knowing the religious outlook and customs of medieval Tibetans, it is difficult to understand the specifics of the graphic information in the *Atlas,* inasmuch as its subject matter characterizes not only elite spiritual culture and the theoretical thinking of a given historical era but also a mass popular culture with centuries-old traditions.

As a document of graphic art, the *Atlas* refers to that period in the history of Tibet's artistic culture when the theoretical and practical legacy of Indian Buddhist art was fully mastered and on that basis national schools of painting and sculpture were created, with their own original treatises on the theory of art, and also when book graphics and book printing developed significantly, thereby enabling a uniform standard for Tibetan graphic art.

In 1991 the Buryats celebrated the 250th anniversary of the official recognition of Buddhism in Transbaikalia. His Holiness the Dalai Lama was the chief guest of this ceremony. As Tibetan Buddhism undergoes a renewal in Russia, along with other spiritual and healing traditions, it is particularly timely to note how this series of paintings stands not only as a testament to religious and aesthetic traditions but to the original cultural traditions of which it is the heart. As a priceless document of Tibetan culture, it offers an integrated and unified view of the world in which body, intellect, and spirit are one.

N. D. Bolsokhoeva and K. M. Gerasimova

Translated from the Russian by Marion Schwartz, with Catherine Fitzpatrick

NOTES

1. As reported by Zhabon to his colleague, D. B. Badlaeva.
2. See A. F. Gammerman and B. V. Semichov, *Slovar' tibetsko-latino-russkikh nazvanii lekarstvennogo rastitel'nogo syr'ia, primeniaemogoBlue Beryltibetsoi meditsine* (Ulan-Ude, 1963), p. 6. [Regarding Baradin, his name appears frequently in John Snelling's account of Tibetan Buddhism in Buryatia. Along with Agvan Dorzhiev, he attempted in the early years a reconciliation (or at least accomodation) between Buddhism and Bolshevism, but nevertheless was one of between four and five hundred orientalists liquidated in the Stalinist purges; he was shot in 1937. See *Buddhism in Russia,* p. 248.—Ed.]
3. Snelling, *Buddhism in Russia,* p. 233.
4. This second version is set forth by P. B. Baldanzhapov in *K izucheniiu istochnikov indo-tibetskoi meditsiny. Materialy po izucheniiu istochnikov traditsionnoi sistemy indo-tibetskoi meditsiny* (Novosibirsk, 1982), p. 15. Baldanzhapov draws upon survey data.
5. Pubaev, R. E. and G. Tsybikov. *G. Ts. Tsybikov: Izbrannye trudy,* vol. 1. (Novosibirsk, 1981), p. 8.
6. Some of these former students of Sunuev, the seventy-year-old lamas Numa Bazarov, Dashi Tsybigmitov, and Baldan Dashiyev told this story in the 1970s.
7. Pubaev, R. E. *Avgan Dorzhiev: Natsionalno-osvoboditelnoe dvizhenie buryatskogo naroda.* (Ulan-Ude, 1989), p. 94.
8. *Buddizm: Slovar'.* (Moscow, 1992), p. 117.
9. Gerasimova, K. M. *Obnovlenchieskoe dvizhenie buryatskogo lamaistskogo dokhovenstva.* (Ulan-Ude, 1964), pp. 144–45, 147–48.
10. Dorzhiev's letter and last testament to his close relative, S. D. Dylykov, was written on September 1, 1936, in the village of Olgino. He wrote: "Finally, I hope that the USSR People's Commissariat of Foreign Affairs [the Soviet foreign ministry] will create for you all the necessary conditions to fulfill your obligations after my death, in the ownership, management, and use of my personal property and real estate at your discretion as

well as the management of the affairs of the Tibetan-Mongolian Mission, to watch over the integrity and preservation of the Buddhist temple with the buildings attached to it and to keep the funds intended for travel to Tibet, including the trip of an official representative of Tibet or a special decision of the Soviet government about the support of an expedition to Tibet, in which you, Dylykov Sandzhe Dantsykovich, must also take part." *(Stranitsy iz zhizni Avgana Dorzhieva: Arkhivnyye dokumenty.* (Ulan-Ude, 1993), p. 114.

11. Gefter, M. Stalinsim, *50/50: Opyt slovrya novogo myshleniya.* (Moscow, 1989), p. 385.
12. Pubaev, R. E. *Agvan Dorzhiev,* p. 50.
13. Badlaeva, D. B. "Nasha pamyat," *Muzey i kraevedenie: problemy istorii i kiltury narodov Buryatii.* (Ulan-Ude, 1993), pp. 9–10.
14. Gumilev, L. N. *Staroburyatskaya zhivopis.* (Moscow, 1975), p. 6.
15. A set of this *Atlas* was published by Galart publishers in 1994. See *Atlas tibetskoi meditsiny: Svod illiustratsii k tibetskomu meditsinskomu traktatu XVII veka "Goluboi berill."* Introductory essays by N. D. Bolsokhoeva, D. B. Dashiev, V. S. Dylykova-Parfionovich, K. M. Gerasimova, L. E. Miall, and T. V. Sergeeva. *Atlas* text translated by T. A. Aseeva, N. D. Bolsokhoeva, T. G. Bukhasheeva, and D. B. Dashiev. Explanatory text to the *Atlas* compiled on the basis of research on the *Four Tantras* and the *Lapis Lazuli* by Yu. M. Parfionovich. Senior editor for the articles by N. D. Bolsokhoeva, K. M. Gerasimova, and D. B. Dashiev, R. E. Pubaev. Scientific editor of the section devoted to medicinal plants and indexer, D. Yu. Butkus. Compiler of glossaries, V. S. Dylkova-Parfionovich. Scientific editor, Yu. M. Parfionovich.
16. Painting 62, which is missing, has drawings illustrating the correct preparation for the study of urine, what the vessel for the urine should be like, and how urine is formed in the organism.
17. Translated from the Sanskrit, beryl means "lapis lazuli"; however, in Tibetan literature there are mentions of yellow, white, and blue beryl *(lapis lazuli),* and the same is true in the titles of the fundamental treatises of the leading theoretician of medieval Tibet, Sangye Gyamtso: the *White Beryl,* the *Yellow Beryl,* and the *Lapis Lazuli [Blue Beryl].* There is a belief that the radiance of the beryl stone chases away diseases that have settled in a person's organism.
18. K. Lange, *Die Regent Sains-rgyas rgya-mtaho (1653–1705).* (Berlin, 1970).
19. Today, scholars have several editions of the Tibetan text of the *Lapis Lazuli,* including the Aginsk edition, published on Russian paper made by the Sumkin factory, which is distinguished by the precision and clarity of its printing. In the 1970s, this commentary was published in full in India and in the People's Republic of China in the form of a European-style bound book.
20. The M. N. Khangalov Museum houses a *Book of Tangyur.*
21. *Tibetan Medical Thangkas of the Four Medical Tantras.* Translator and compiler of the original edition, *Byams-pa Phrin las,* Wang Lei. English translator and annotator, Cai Jingfeng. (Lhasa, 1988).
22. Apti is a shortened form of his full Sanskrit name, Buddha Apti.
23. The five major sciences (Buddhist philosophy, logic, medicine, grammar, and Buddhism) and the five minor sciences (the technology of crafts, the theory of poetry, linguistics, astrology, and choreography) comprise the foundation of a Buddhist classical education.
24. The Soviet specialists A. F. Gammerman, a pharmacologist, and B. V. Semichev, a Tibetologist, began their study of Tibetan medicine back in the late 1920s and early 1930s. They first came across the *Atlas of Tibetan Medicine* in 1958, when they learned of its existence from Gerasimova. They then became more familiar with it, utilizing the archives of the History Museum of Buryatia in Ulan-Ude. Gammerman and Semichev, authors of the *Dictionary of Tibetan-Latin-Russian Terms for Medicinal Plants Used in Tibetan Medicine,* made use in their work only of those paintings in the *Atlas* that referred to medicinal plants, which they proposed publishing as a second illustrated section of the dictionary (copies of the medicinal plants from the *Atlas* were executed by the artists A. Okladnikov, T. Rud, and E. Nevolina, but were not published). Here it is important to note that the section on medicinal plants in the *Atlas* comprises 540 drawings of medicinal plants whose names are included in the published dictionary. A second group comprises 120 names of plants not included in the dictionary, 67 of which have been identified either precisely or approximately, and 53 of which remain unidentified.

The information in the *Four Tantras,* the *Lapis Lazuli,* and the *Atlas of Tibetan Medicine* was used in cultural studies for the first time in 1967 by Gerasimova, when she was researching Tibetan and Mongolian sources on the theory of Buddhist art for her monograph, *Documents in the Aesthetic Thought of the East: The Tibetan Canon of Proportions.*

The Buddha's Art of Healing: Catalogue

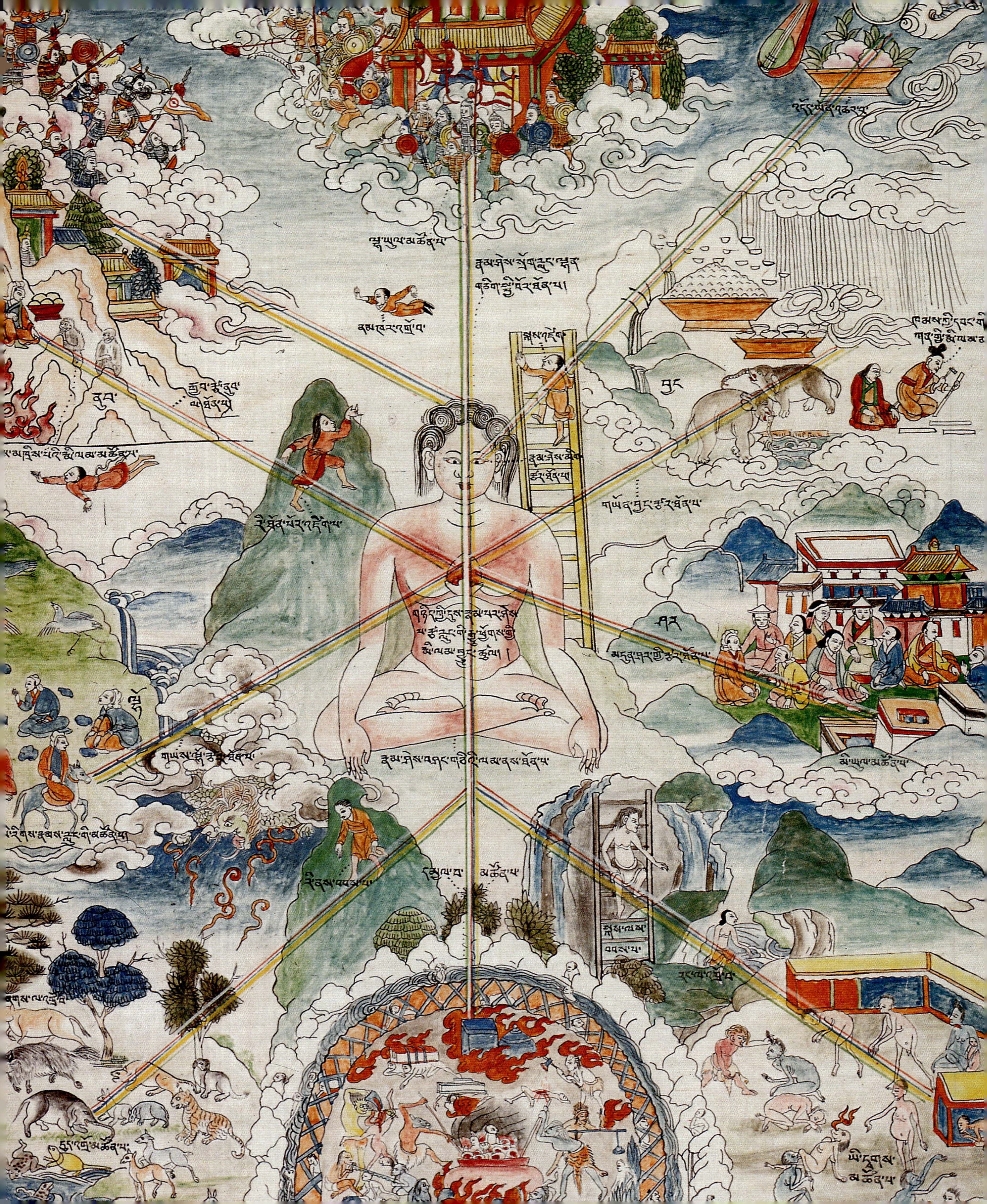

The Painted Guide to the Teachings of Tibetan Medicine

The forty Tibetan paintings reproduced here stem from a series of seventy-nine created as illustrations of the seventeenth-century commentary on the most fundamental treatise of Tibetan medicine, the *Four Tantras* or *Gyushi*. The words of the *Four Tantras* are presented as those of the Healing Buddha, offered to a gathering of listeners through the intermediary of his emanation, the sage whose name is Wisdom of Knowledge. Only one of these listeners, the sage Born of the Spirit (Manasija), fully understood the teachings and committed them to writing, after which they were transmitted through an uninterrupted lineage of masters, first in India and then in Tibet.

The Tibetan view of the origin of dreams finds connections between the images in dreams, the energies of the body, and the realms of the spirit. Those of the gods are pictured above; those of hell, below (detail, pl. 14).

These works of art that constitute the *Atlas of Tibetan Healing* bear eloquent witness not only to the Tibetan Science of Healing as systematized in the *Four Tantras* but also to its profound history, embodied in the line of masters who may be seen in the upper registers of many of these paintings (see plates 1–8, 13, and 19). Undertaken at the impetus of Sangye Gyamtso, the regent of the Fifth Dalai Lama, these paintings spring from the same didactic vision that distinguishes the regent's entire medical legacy. It was he who in fact determined that they should be created, conceived of their extraordinary scope, and supervised their realization. Great lengths were gone to for the verification of the previously existing iconographic elements on which the works in part depend. For example, to verify the accuracy of the topographical lines indicative of the location of the underlying organs (see plates 5–7, 9, and 10), the regent took Tendzin Norbuchen, head of the painting corps of the Potala Palace, away from his task of directing its decoration, dispatching him instead to the funerary sites to make anatomical drawings after cadavers which, in keeping with the traditional Tibetan practice, had been thrown to the vultures. This quest for realism was carried out also in relation to the hundreds of objects illustrated in the *materia medica* (see plates 24–27); the court painters drew directly from samples gathered from all regions of the country, and according to information provided by people consulted by the regent. When the series was finally completed, in 1703 at the latest, it literally illustrated the entire contents of the *Four Tantras* and its commentary, the *Blue Beryl*. Its grand synthetic compositions, all bearing captions, and the hundreds of small figures, each of them accompanied by a concise inscription from the text, testify to the pedagogic ambitions and novelty of the finished work. "This unprecedented series of paintings," the regent wrote, "was created so that anyone, from the child to the scholar, could perceive the entire contents as easily as he perceives the appearance of a myrobalan fruit held in the palm of the hand."

The images fulfill a double mission. Some of the paintings, with their anatomical figures or illustrations of medicinal plants, supplement the text, providing graphic indications of topographical reference points, for example, or visual depictions of the *materia medica*. The others, covered with hundreds of tiny vignettes that follow one another across the horizontal

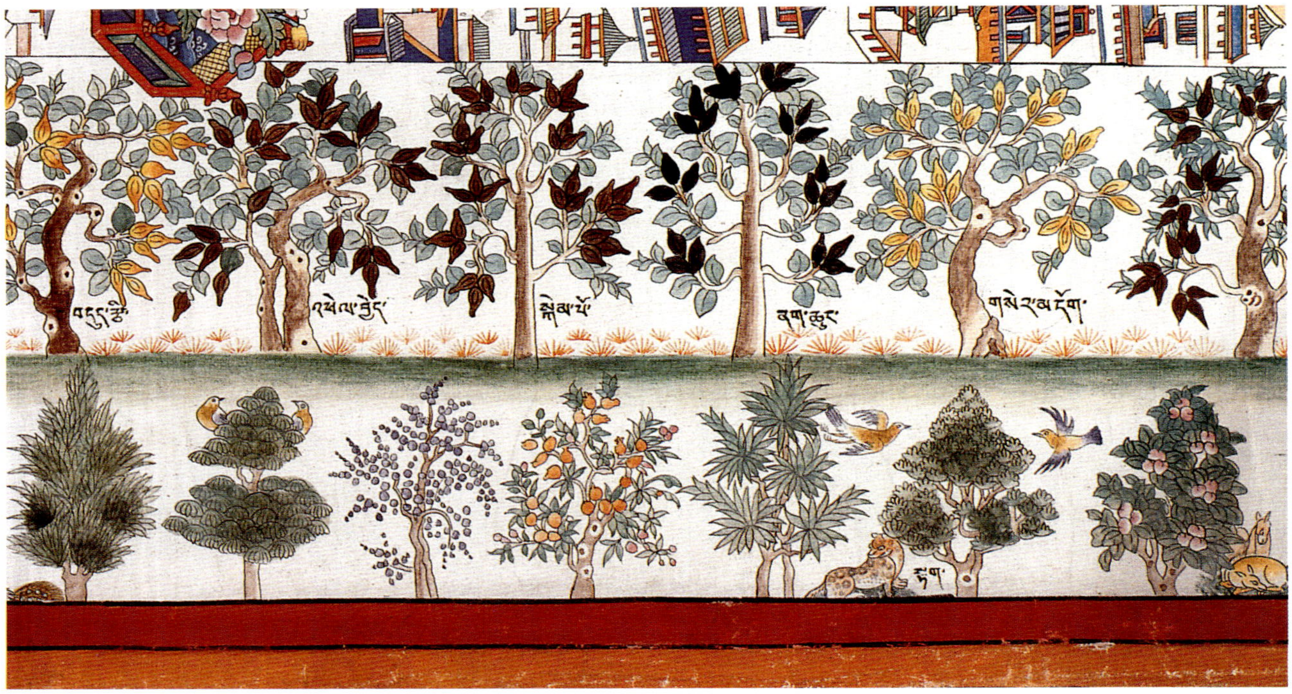

Myrobalan trees (detail, pl. 1). The myrobalan fruit is a panacea for all illnesses, and as such may be seen in the first painting in this volume, in which it is held within the Healing Buddha's right hand in a gesture of generosity.

registers in the manner of a comic strip, offer merely a summary paraphrase of the texts and thus add no new information. Most of the paintings of the series are subdivided by horizontal lines into bands where drawings run from left to right and from top to bottom in the order in which their subjects are mentioned in the *Blue Beryl.* The successive vignettes are usually single elements, such as a human figure or a plant, but sometimes also comprise small architectural or landscape scenes. They were created not only to provide information but also to capture one's attention. The painters provided an infinite variation in the attitudes and movements of the figures, with a vitality and zest that Tibetan artists knew how to instill into narrative painting.

The series was most effective as a teaching tool of Tibetan medicine. From the eighteenth century onward, the series was often reproduced and widely disseminated. Reproduced either individually or as a complete series, the paintings have been copied on canvas, painted on the walls of medical colleges, and even printed on paper. Some of the paintings traveled quite far; the ones presented here are from a nearly complete series (seventy-six from the original seventy-nine) that reached Buryatia. This series is one of at least three sets known to exist in the world today, along with one other from the summer palace of the Dalai Lama (Norbulingka), now in possession of the Commission for Cultural Relics of the Autonomous Region of Tibet, and another belonging to the School of Medicine and Astrology (Mendzekhang) in Lhasa.

As we have seen, this iconographic series precisely follows the content of the *Blue Beryl* and hence of the *Four Tantras.* Each of the four volumes of this latter treatise treats the same subjects as the others, but more or less deeply and from a different perspective. The medical paintings included here have been selected so as to avoid redundancy and are arranged according to a few major thematic lines that follow one another logically, rather than in strict adherence to their numerical order in the series.

The Tibetan Science of Healing as expounded in the *Four Tantras* cannot be called empirical medicine. On the contrary, it was consciously elaborated as a sophisticated, rationally constructed system, whose parts, whether they derive from empirical experience or theoretical speculation, form a coherent, integrated whole obeying the rules of epistemology and formal logic as well as a limited number of natural laws. The "tree" paintings (see plates 2, 13, and 19), introducing the themes of physiology and physiopathology, diagnosis, and treatment, eloquently illustrate this systematic organization, in which every part has its place within a clearly delineated, coherent whole. They present the various elements of Tibetan medical science in summary form, as pictograms distributed along the branches and on the leaves of the three trees. The successive branchings of each of the trees make visible the logical connections of the constitutive elements, both among themselves and as parts of the whole.

Tibetan medicine shares with Buddhist philosophy a number of fundamental concepts concerning the status of the person and the material nature of the phenomenal world, concepts that differ substantially from the Western orientation. From the Buddhist perspective, the person is a temporary aggregate of five orders of phenomena in permanent flux: form, sensation, discrimination, volition, and consciousness. Form manifests itself in the anatomy of the body and also in the fluids and humors *(nyes-pas)* that ensure the body's physiological functioning. Most notably, the Cartesian dualism of the West is absent: Tibetan medicine does not recognize a radical opposition between the mind and the body. Instead, mind and body constitute a single totality in which the somatic and the psychic interact with one another.

This difference has profound consequences in relation to views of disease. For example, there are a number of systems for the classification of diseases. While one of them does employ the two pathological categories of physical and psychic disorders, this is simply a matter of convenience. This difference also must color our understanding of the humoral theory of the body, which is so important in Tibetan medicine and is touched on by all authors of the present volume. The reciprocal equilibrium of the three humors is expressed within individual temperaments having both biological and psychological features. Humoral disorders can cause emotional and psychic disorders as well as somatically manifested illnesses (see plate 39). Conversely, pathogenic factors include not only physical causes such as food and toxic substances, but also those of a psychic, ethical, and even interpersonal nature. It should be noted that of the three humors—*mkhris-pa, bad-kan,* and *rlung*—it is the latter that plays the greatest role in integrating the body and mind.

Not only are body and mind one. The person is seen in relation to the entire ecological environment, and this relationship is given very precise definition. Everything in the material world, however subtle and whether living or not, derives from a combination of some or all of the five elements: earth, water, fire, wind, and space. This view derives from ancient, commonly shared Indian ideas, and was introduced to Tibet through Buddhist literature, as well as through translations of Ayurvedic medical texts. The body itself is seen as an aggregate of the five elements, which combine in variable proportions to form its constitutive parts. Consciousness is the centralizing principle for all sensory information and the seat of discursive thought. Underpinned by a subconscious principle conditioned by past actions, consciousness transmigrates

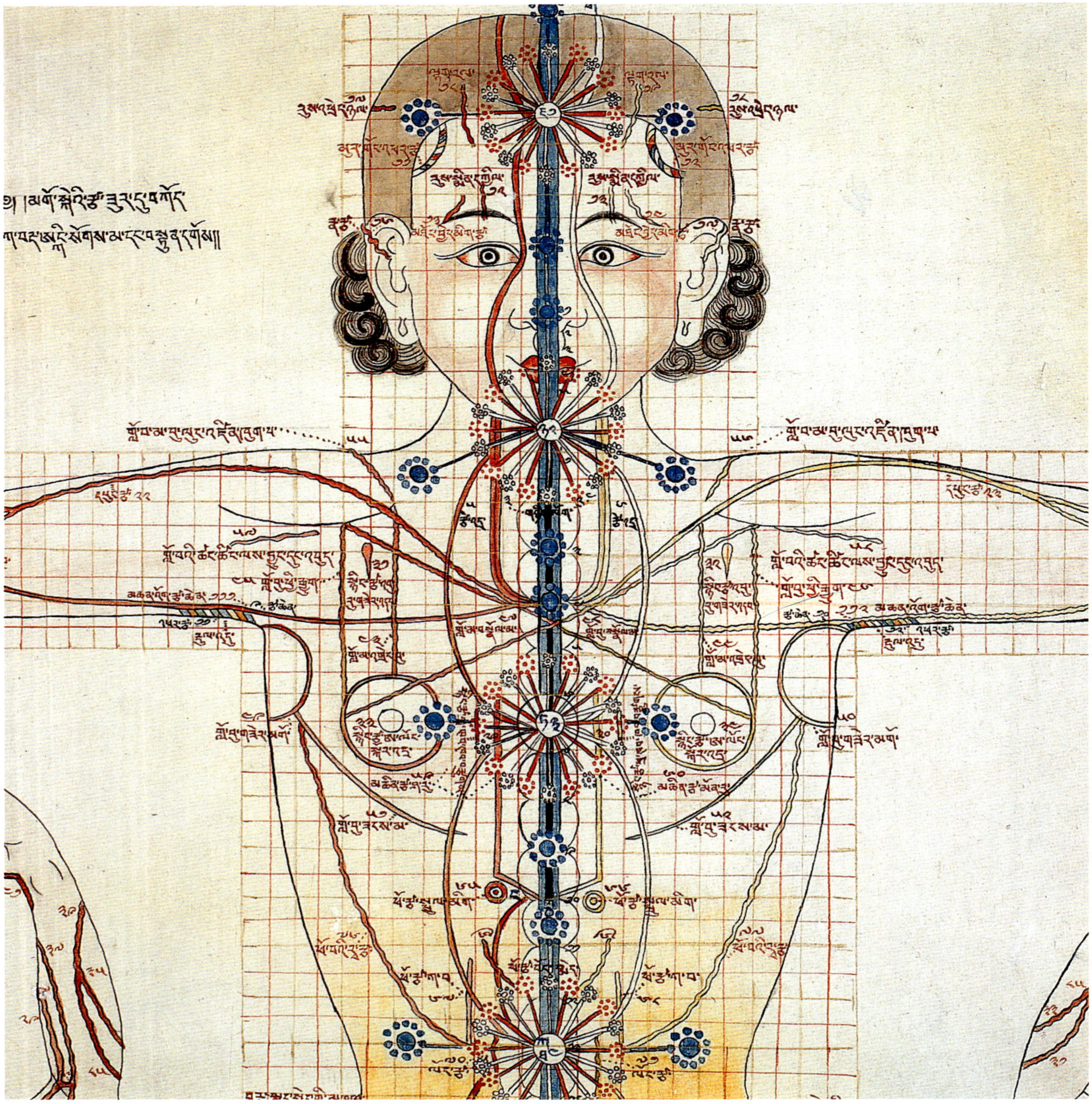

A detail (pl. 6) illustrating the more than five hundred channels that integrate the mind and body. Of four basic types, they intersect to form *chakras.*

from one existence to another when the elements that make up the body come apart at the moment of death.

Within the living body, the elements combine in various proportions to form the seven bodily constituents: blood, flesh, fat, bone, marrow, reproductive fluid, and nutritional "essence" from ingested food. These form a substratum for the three humors, which carry out the various physiologic functions. *Bad-kan,* whose nature is that of the element water, carries out the body's mechanical functions, such as cohesion and support. *Mkhris-pa,* associated with fire, produces body heat and digestion, likened to a cooking of food. Its active nature contrasts with the passivity of *bad-kan.* The *rlung* humor, which shares the nature of wind, displays the latter's characteristic mobility. It has a special status in manifesting as the "vital breath" and in causing the humor to expand out from its usual location at the beginning of each disease. It is also involved in all bodily functions having to do with movement. It controls sensory perception, as well as psychic activity. Each of these three humors appears in five different and more or less subtle forms, with their own specialized function and distinct location, or seat, in the various tissues, organs, or other parts of the body. The physiological processes performed by these humors during digestion or in the tissues are accompanied by the production of residues, the most important of which are feces, urine, and sweat. The nutritional "essence" from ingested food, blood, the humors, and other fluids such as the metabolic fluids from which the tissues are built, circulate in different types of channels linked together as a network in the body.

Each humor presents characteristics that derive from a longer list of qualities describing substances in general. The different sensible qualities of substances are said to result from the particular combination of the elements that constitute the substances themselves. The most important of these sensible qualities are the tastes and the potencies, which relate to the activities of the substances according to a general law that maintains that a given quality will excite all substances presenting this same quality and, conversely, will inhibit those that present the opposite quality. The same may be said of the characteristics of the humors. Hence *bad-kan* is considered oily, cold, heavy, dull, stable, and sticky. *Mkhris-pa* is oily, sharp, hot, light, fetid, purgative, and moistening. *Rlung* is rough, light, cold, subtle, firm, and mobile. The distribution of those characteristics among the three humors is clearly not arbitrary, but reflects in large measure an empirical observation of the body fluids, considered the principles of biological activity. Among the characteristics of the humors, the hot/cold pair predominates. *Bad-kan* shares the cold nature of the moon and *mkhris-pa* the hot nature of the sun. *Rlung* is seen either as cold in nature or as neutral.

The humors fulfill essential functions in the body, and, so long as they are maintained in a state of balance relative to each individual constitution, they confer life and health. Illness, then, is simply the manifestation of imbalance among these humors and reflects an inherent potential of the humors themselves, one that remains latent until triggered by a pathogenic cause. In the *Four Tantras* the notion is expressed in the following way: "Suffering is attached to a being even in good health, just as the shadow follows the bird even when it is flying in the sky." The humors are therefore the primary causes of illnesses, which arise when triggered by any of four categories of immediate causes: food, lifestyle, the seasons, and evil spirits. Toxic agents, errors in treatment, and wounds are also considered immediate causes. But given the importance of the Indo-Tibetan notion of karma, the effects of negative actions of the past are also likely to be invoked in the etiology of disease. The immediate causes are believed to provoke pathological imbalances either by exciting the humors through the affinities of their shared sensible qualities, or by suppressing them through the antagonism of their opposite qualities. Thus foods that are too heavy and sweet, or a lifestyle that is too sedentary and idle can bring on, particularly at the end of winter, a pathogenic excess of *bad-kan,* for it shares the same sensible qualities. The humors themselves are said to arise from more remote causes, namely the three poisons of desire, hatred, and delusion that according to the most ancient Buddhist notions enslave beings to

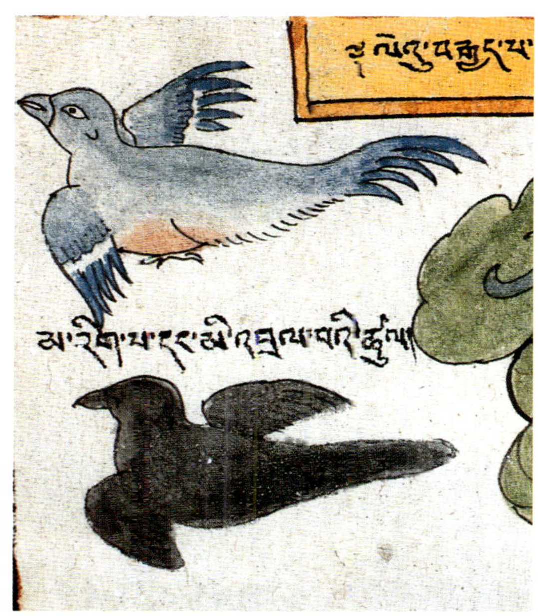

In the Tibetan system, illness is part and parcel of health. Even in good health, suffering is attached to being, "just as the shadow follows the bird even when it is flying in the sky" (detail, pl. 12).

the endless cycle of rebirths. These three moral poisons have their own final cause—fundamental ignorance.

Even though a pathogenic imbalance can theoretically result from either an increase or a decrease in one or more of the humors, the pathology described by Tibetan physiopathological theory is primarily that of excess. Under the influence of an immediate cause, the susceptible humor increases and accumulates, at first in the body tissues and residues that are its normal substrata. At this stage, the illness does not yet display clear clinical signs. Renewed contact with the immediate cause brings about an overt arising of the humor already accumulated. Like a rising lake that breaches its dikes, the humor overflows from its usual location and spreads along the pathogenic pathways, or the six "doors of disease": skin, flesh, channels, bones, the five full organs (heart, lungs, liver, kidneys, spleen), and six hollow organs (stomach, gall bladder, small and large intestines, urinary bladder, and reproductive organs). The illness has now declared itself and its signs are clearly manifest on the surface of the body, as well as in the pulse or the urine. The *Four Tantras* also mentions the fifteen paths of diffusion, five for each of the three humors in its pathogenic state. These paths, which seem to represent a different model from that of the pathogenic pathways, are body tissues, residues or excreta, sense organs, full organs, and hollow organs.

Theoretically, clinical signs merely manifest the qualities of humors that have become pathogenic as well as the repercussions of their imbalances in the structures where they have their "seat."

Diagnostic Techniques in Tibetan Medicine

Diagnosis is defined as the outcome of a process of logical inference made possible by the necessary and sufficient relations that unite the clinical signs to the illness. That is, inference is a rational process that infers something you do not see from something you can perceive. For example: when you see smoke on a mountain from afar you can infer the existence of a fire you do not see, or from a given symptom or a set of symptoms you can infer the existence of a given disease. The inference leads to certain conclusions only if the sign (smoke) and what it signifies (fire) are linked by a relation both necessary (no fire if there is no smoke) and sufficient (smoke does not need the presence of other signs to indicate the existence of fire). In Tibetan medicine, the physician's task is to confront a range of information obtained through three of the five senses—hearing, touch, and vision, each the basis of one of the three elements of the traditional examination: inquiry, feeling the pulse, and observation, particularly of the tongue and urine.

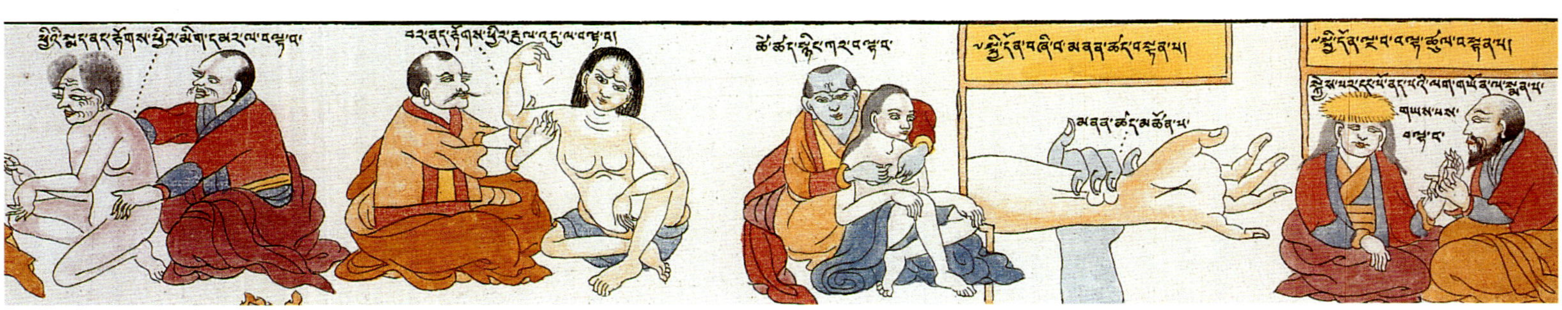

Western doctors are intrigued by the precision of Tibetan pulse diagnosis, a central technique of Tibetan medicine. Here the proper placement of the fingers is shown (detail, pl. 15).

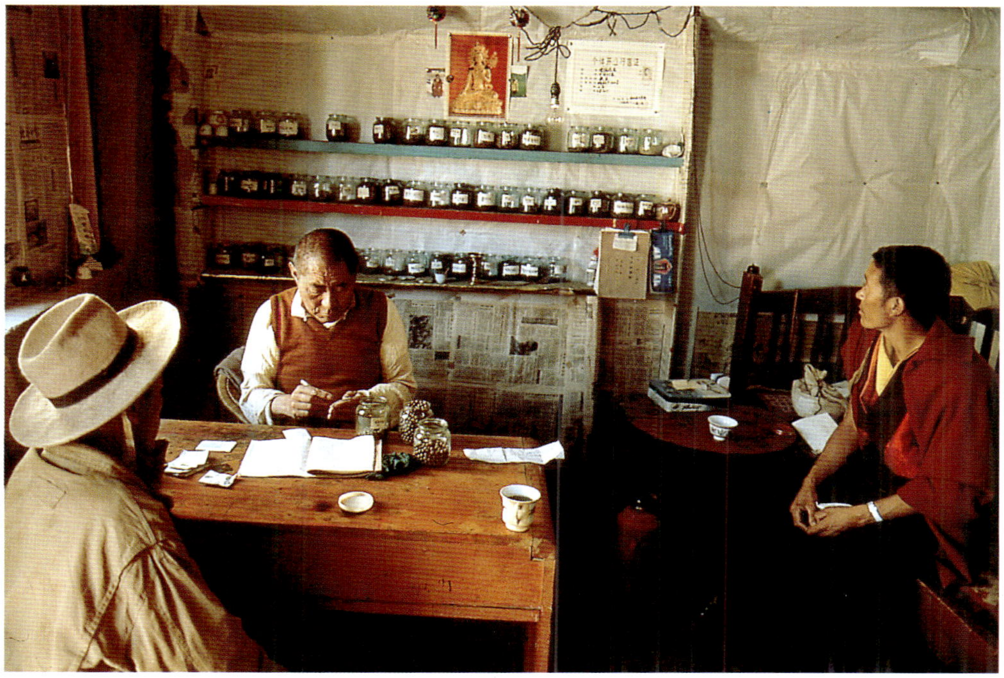

Left: Patients consult a doctor in Ganzi, Tibet.

Below: A Tibetan nun suffering from the continuing effects of political torture is treated by Tenzin Choedrak, senior physician of His Holiness the Dalai Lama.

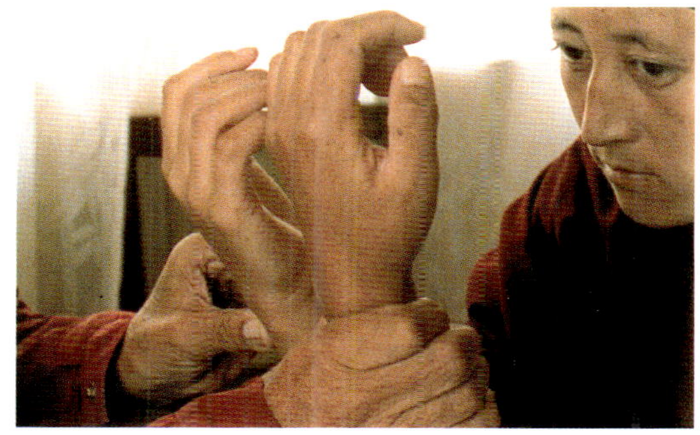

An examination normally begins with an interview during which the physician inquires into the patient's eating habits, lifestyle, environment, and so on in order to discover the immediate causes of the illness. The physician also asks about the patient's current habits and behaviors in order to determine which of them soothe or aggravate the complaint. The process is similar to the Western one of "taking the history."

Palpation of the pulse is the indispensable element in the diagnostic practice of Tibetan physicians and is favored over all others. In Tibet, the image of the practitioner reading the patient's pulse is as emblematic of medicine there as was, in medieval Europe, that of the physician in the act of gazing at a vial of urine. Pulse diagnosis seems to have been borrowed from China, with some modification in the details of the procedure. Usually after a brief interview with the patient, the physician begins by placing three fingers on the radial arteries of the right and left wrists of the patient, who faces the doctor with elbows bent and forearms extended. Under each of his three fingers on each side, the doctor checks the pulse in relation to the condition of a part of the body (upper, middle, and lower) and that of two organs: a full organ under the upper edge of the finger or a hollow organ under the lower edge. By noting the particular characteristics of the pulse—its frequency, force, form, speed, tension, firmness, and so on—the physician is supposed to diagnose not only the type of humoral imbalance afflicting the patient but also its location in the body and the specific illness in question. According to the *Four Tantras,* the examination of the pulse can also serve as a method of divination (see plates 15 and 16) used in determining, for example, the outcome of business transactions, the likelihood of receiving visitors, spirit interference, or matters of marriage and children.

The practice of uroscopy, or observation of the urine, relies primarily on the sense of vision. As a practical matter, this procedure has fallen out of favor, largely because of the difficulty of performing it during the course of a modern office visit. Indeed, for a proper uroscopic examination, the urine should be collected on the patient's awakening, before he has had anything to eat, and it should be examined immediately. This sophisticated and specifically Tibetan technique has no equivalents in other Asian medical traditions. The fresh urine is examined while still warm, and then at several stages as it cools. The examination takes into account not only the color of the urine and the suspension of elements in it, but also the vapor, bubbles, and floating matter, and changes as it cools. Like pulse examination, uroscopy provides both general information about the relevant pathogenic humors and more precise indications as to the locations involved and the particular type of disease. Like pulse examination, uroscopy can serve as a method of divination.

Treatment in Tibetan Medicine

Treatment involves four types of "antagonists" or "antidotes": lifestyle, diet, medicines, and external therapy. As the general term *antagonist* indicates, therapy is based on the principle of opposites. Generally speaking, an excess of a particular humor is countered by opposing it with a treatment having contrary qualities. The four types of antagonists are listed in order of increasing strength and progressive application, the stronger antagonists generally being used later and added to the milder ones in response to more aggravated conditions. No clear distinction is made between foods and drugs; it is thought that they work in the same way. The sensible qualities of the therapeutic substances, whether foods or drugs, are what give them their particular biological effects. These qualities, which are divided among several categories—tastes, potencies, post-digestive tastes, and so on—are themselves determined by the respective proportions of the elements that compose any given substance. Among all the natural properties of substances, the five tastes—acidic, salty, bitter, hot, and astringent—play a preeminent role. They can occur in isolation or in combination, each one being determined by the preponderance of two of the five elements.

The biological activity of substances is also explained by another group of eight sensible qualities called potencies, expressed as a series of four pairs of opposites: hot/cold, heavy/light, oily/rough, dull/sharp. These potencies are directly determined by the tastes and indirectly

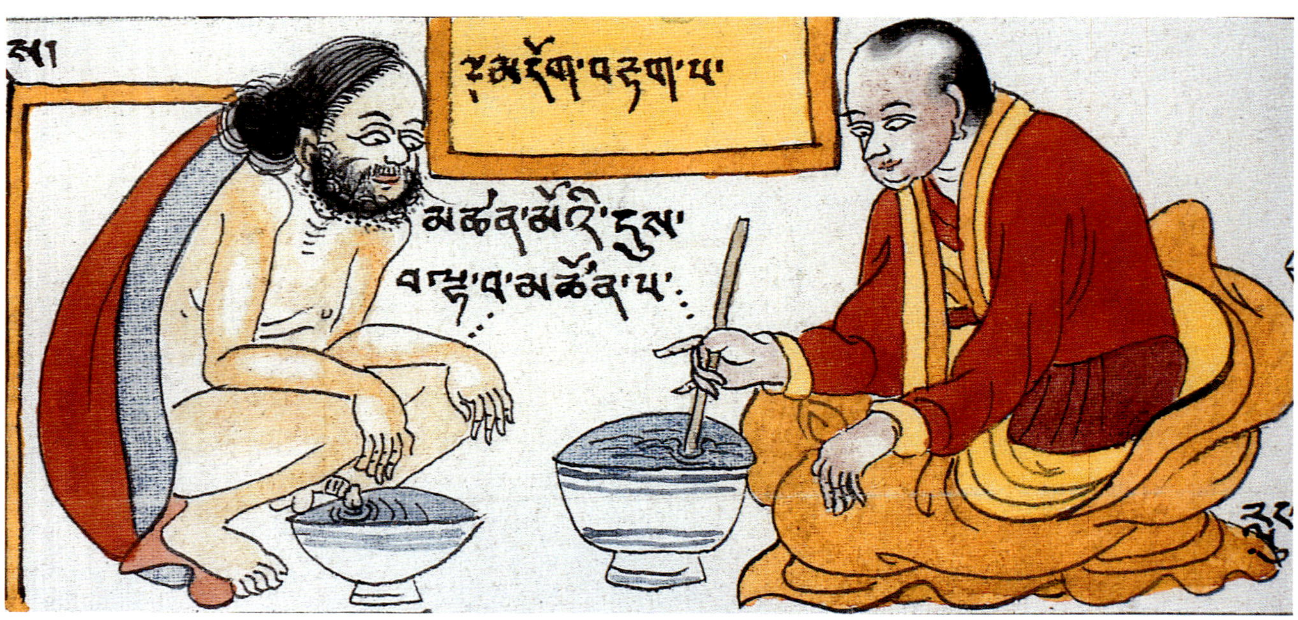

Uroscopy: examining the urine while it is still warm. This diagnostic technique has fallen out of favor, and is one of the most complicated aspects of Tibetan medicine (detail, pl. 18).

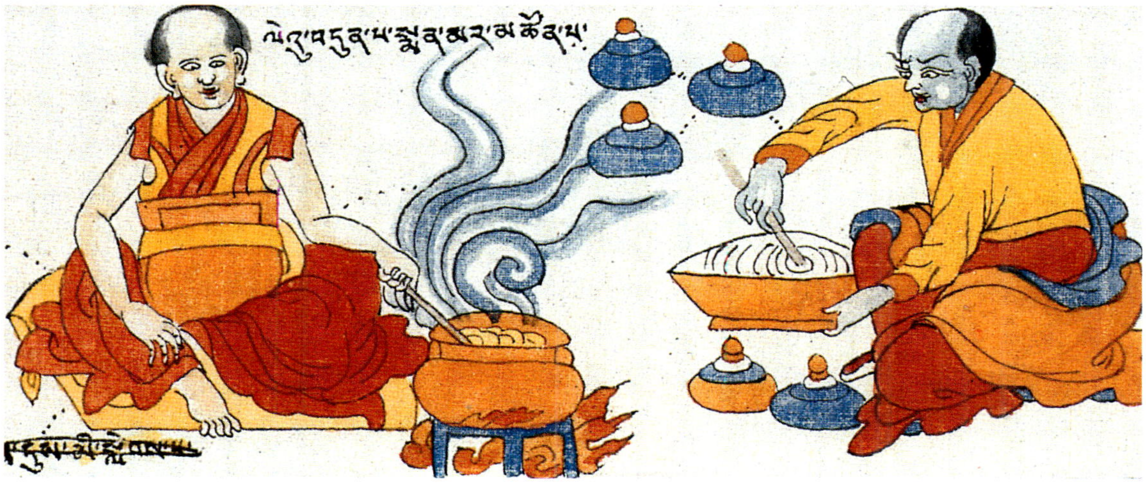

Making the soothing remedies (tranquilizing agents). Within Tibetan pharmacology, many active ingredients work together in methods now being explored by proponents of "complementary" Western medicine (detail, pl. 28).

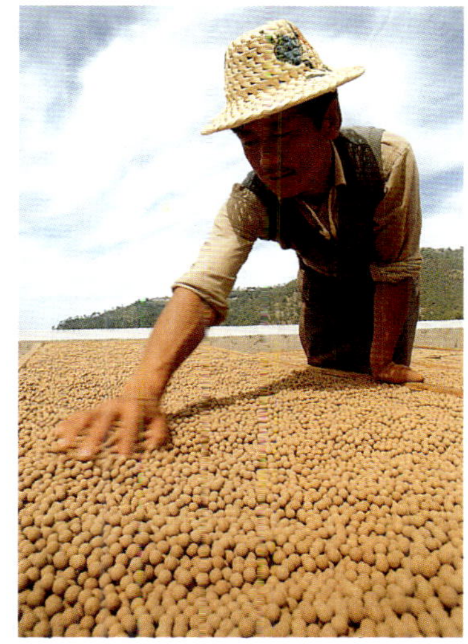

Sorting Tibetan herbal remedies in Dharamsala, India.

by the five elements. Among the eight potencies, hot and cold are considered to be predominant. The eight principle potencies are part of a longer list of seventeen sensible qualities. Once substances are ingested, they are transformed in the digestive process, a fact that accounts for the clinical observation that certain substances do not produce the biological activity their natural tastes might be expected to yield. For this reason, the post-digestive tastes are said to determine their biological activity. Like the Indian Ayurvedic tradition from which it in many respects derives, the Tibetan medical tradition recognizes several levels of pharmaceutical action: natural tastes, potencies, post-digestive tastes of the isolated drugs, and synergistic effects of compound remedies.

Tibetan medicines fall into two major categories: soothing remedies, which work by appeasing the pathogenic humors, and evacuating remedies, whose action is to expel these humors from the body. The soothing remedies restore the pathogenic humor to its proper location and normal level. They comprise ten different kinds: decoctions, medicinal powders, pills, sweet or fat pastes, medicinal butters, concentrates, metallic and mineral ashes, fermented medicinal beverages, gemstone medications, and herbal compounds. The evacuating remedies, or cathartic procedures, eliminate the morbid humor from the organism. They include purgatives, emetics, medicinal snuffs, mild enemas, strong enemas, and cleansing of the channels.

The following passage from the *Four Tantras* demonstrates the idea of progressive application in the use of these different treatments:

> For any disorder one must first prescribe decoctions with sharp and rapid potencies in order to ripen, gather, and isolate the morbid humor. If this method fails then powders should be given. To eliminate the remaining pathogenic factors embedded in the channels, joints, skin, and so forth, sweet or fat pastes should be administered. Finally, in order to strengthen the body and clear the sense organs, medicinal butters are used. Purgation expels blood, bile, and so forth downward. Emetics cast *bad-kan,* poisons, and so forth upward. Snuffs eliminate pathogenic factors that are located in the head and

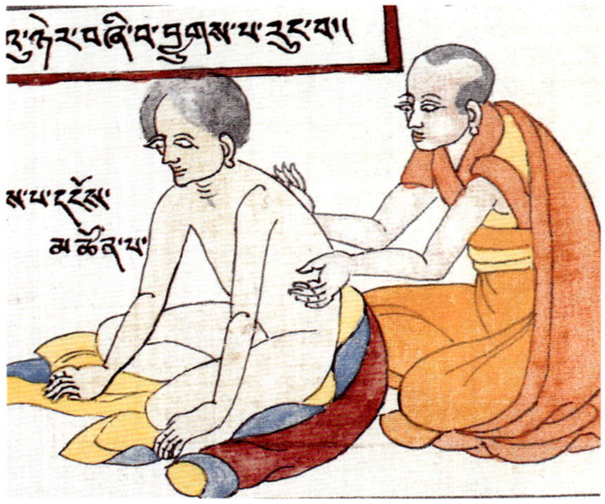

Administering ointments—oils and medicine pastes—employed for such diverse treatments as the reduction of cellulite and the enhancement of memory (detail, pl. 34).

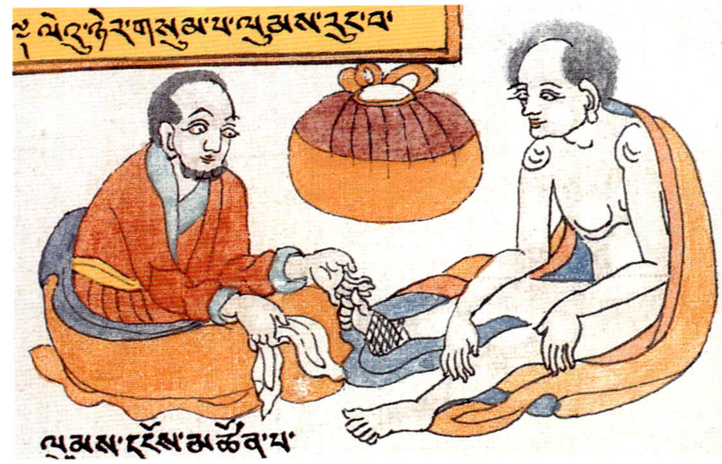

Administering compresses, the most effective painkillers in Tibetan medicine (detail, pl. 34).

> neck. Mild and strong enemas eject disorders from the colon and the small intestine. Finally, purgation of the channels enables one to overcome the disorder when all the preceding methods have failed.

External treatments include those that help rid the body of the residues of pathogenic factors that have proven resistent to treatment through medication. According to the *Four Tantras,* bloodletting eliminates the residues of hot disorders. Moxibustion destroys the force of cold disorders. External applications are indicated when two or three humors in which *bad-kan* predominates are out of balance. When *mkhris-pa* predominates, hot compresses and medicinal baths are used. Oily ointments are used when *rlung* predominates. Finally, minor surgery is employed when the disorder has not responded to the preceding treatments. Such surgery includes cauterization, excision or wounds, traumatology, removal of foreign bodies like arrowheads, evacuation of abcesses or collected fluid, removal of certain tumors, or even minor eye surgery on cataracts. In contemporary Tibetan medical practice, treatment consists mainly of the administration of powders and pills. The only external therapeutic technique that is regularly used is moxibustion.

The relationship of the paintings that follow to the *Four Tantras* and the *Blue Beryl* has been dealt with in my previous essay and in the essay by Bolsokhoeva and Gersimova in this volume. Dr. Bradley's descriptions of these works of art below are cursory and simplified, an introductory gloss of physiological and pathological concepts that often have no direct correspondence in the context of modern Western medicine. It is hoped that the reader, to whatever degree, may perceive Tibetan medicine as the fruit of an admirable effort to integrate empirical observation with a form of rational theoretical speculation. In keeping with the Buddhist philosophy on which it is based, Tibetan medicine considers each person, whether healthy or sick, in the totality of his dimensions—physical and spiritual—in his relation to others and to the world.

FERNAND MEYER

Translated from the French by Arthur Denner

THE PAINTINGS

Commentaries by Tamdin S. Bradley

1. The Palace of the Healing Buddha

Homage to the Buddha Vaiduryaprabha,
Transcendent One acting with compassion for all living beings,
The mere hearing of whose name offers sanctuary from the
sufferings of inferior existences,
Spiritual Master of medicine, dispelling diseases caused by the three poisons—
Desire, Hatred, and Delusion.

—*Buddhist prayer, translated by Gyurme Dorje*

This painting shows the Master of Remedies, the Healing Buddha, teaching to his retinue in the medicinal City of Irresistible Beauty, believed to be located in the land of Oddiyana, in northwestern India. The city is square; it has four gates.

To the south is the Piercing Mountain, dominated by the power of the sun. Here conditions are right for growing medicinal plants of a hot and sharp potency, such as pomegranate, pepper, and cinnamon. These have a hot, sour, and salty taste, and cure all diseases of a cold nature.

To the north is the Snow Mountain, dominated by the power of the moon. Here conditions are right for growing medicinal plants of a cooling potency, such as white sandalwood, camphor, eaglewood, gentian, and licorice. They have a bitter, sweet, and astringent taste, and cure all diseases of a hot nature.

To the east is the Fragrant Mountain, dominated equally by the powers of the sun and moon. Here conditions are right for growing many varieties of the myrobalan fruit, the most powerful being the "victorious myrobalan," panacea for all diseases.

To the west is the Malaya Mountain, rich with rocks and minerals such as the five calcites that cure all chronic diseases; the five bitumens; and the five hot springs. Here grow the six primary ingredients of Tibetan medicine: nutmeg, clove, cardamom, saffron, bamboo pith, and cubeb.

All medicinal ingredients are grown on these four mountains.

Within the city lies the Healing Buddha's palace, made and decorated with precious stones that can cure the 404 kinds of disease. In the center of the palace sits the Healing Buddha, on a throne made of wish-fulfilling jewels. He is surrounded by a retinue of gods, sages, Hindu divinities, and Buddhist disciples, each understanding and interpreting his teachings.

The Buddha is blue, the color of lapis lazuli. His radiance can cure the three poisons of desire, hatred, and delusion. His right hand is held out in a gesture of generosity, cradling the myrobalan fruit. His left hand holds a begging bowl filled with a nectar that can heal all disease.

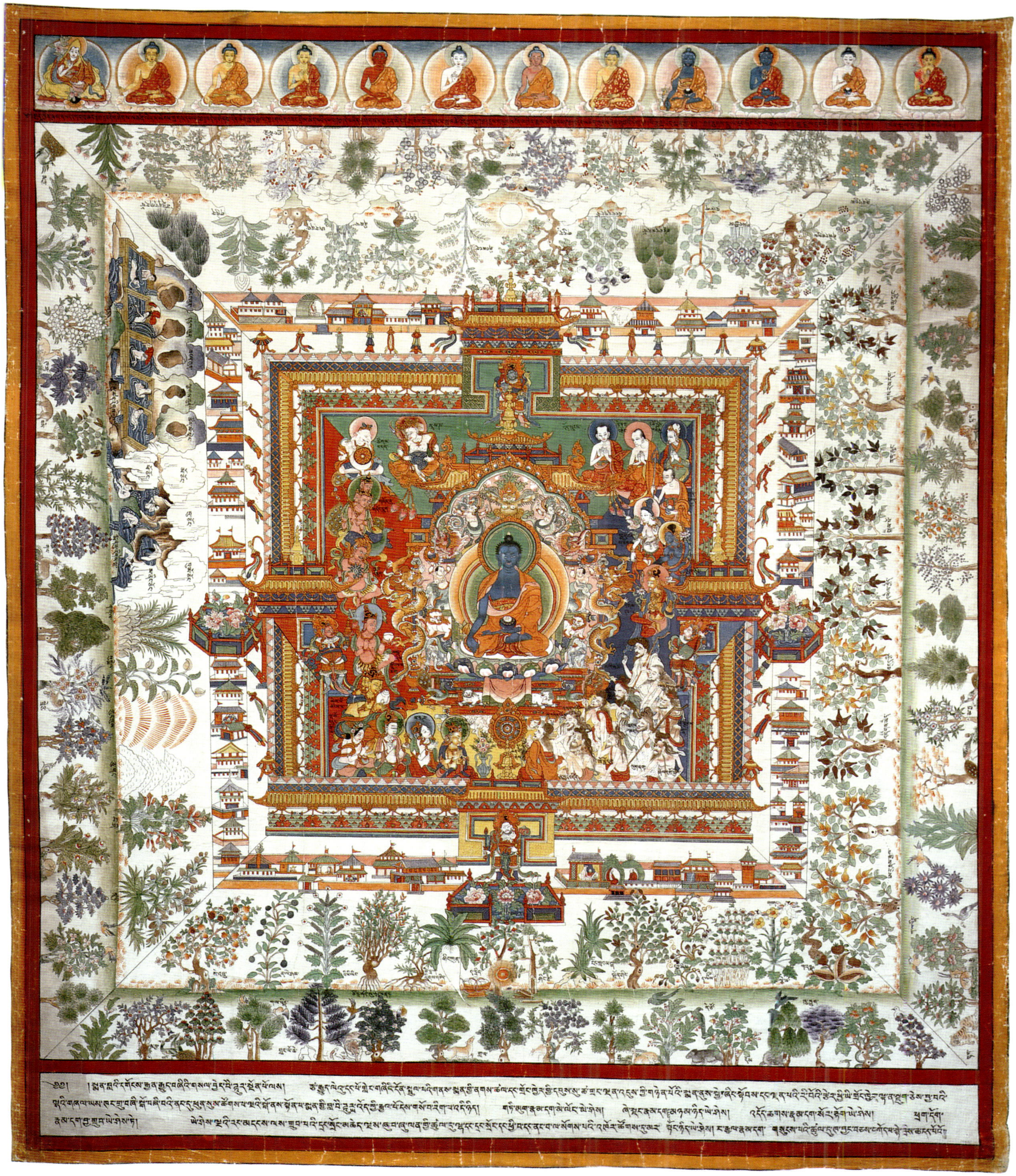

2. The Tree of Health and Disease

1. The Root Tantra;
2. The Explanatory Tantra;
3. The Instructional Tantra; and
4. The Subsequent Tantra.

These four tantras together contain 156 chapters with 5,900 verses dealing with the following eight branches of medicine:

1. the body (includes embryology, anatomy, physiology, pathology, pharmacology);
2. pediatrics;
3. gynecology;
4. disorders caused by spirits;
5. disorders from wounds inflicted by weapons;
6. toxicology;
7. rejuvenation; and
8. aphrodisiacs.

The tantras are composed in the form of a dialogue between the teacher, Vidyajñana, and the student, Manasija, both of whom were emanations of the Healing Buddha. In this painting they are portrayed on the far left of the register at the top.

This painting illustrates the Root Tantra. From the root of the tree grow two trunks; to the left are the mind and body in a healthy state, and to the right are the mind and body in an unhealthy state.

The healthy trunk has three branches.

The lower branch contains the three *nyes-pas* [humors]: *rlung* (pronounced "loong"; air/movement), *mkhris-pa* (pronounced "treeba"; fire/heat), and *bad-kan* (pronounced "baygan"; fluid/water/earth).[1] *Rlung* is the subtle flow of energy that assists the workings of the mind, body, and speech. *Mkhris-pa* is the heat that regulates bodily temperature and aids digestion. *Bad-kan* helps sustain bodily fluids. On the lower branch, the blue leaves are the five subdivisions of *rlung;* the yellow leaves are the five subdivisions of *mkhris-pa;* and the white leaves are the five subdivisions of *bad-kan.* The middle branch shows the seven bodily constituents: nutritional "essence" from ingested food; blood; flesh; fat; bone; marrow; and the reproductive fluids. The upper branch shows the excretory functions as the three leaves of defecation, urination, and perspiration.

The twenty-five leaves on the three branches show how important it is for the three *nyes-pas,* seven bodily constituents, and three excretory functions to be in balance. We are then able to enjoy good health and longevity, symbolized by the two flowers in the upper portion of the painting. These blossoms represent the fulfillment of our need to practice a spiritual life and to accumulate wealth and happiness, symbolized by the three fruits.

The unhealthy trunk has nine branches and sixty-three leaves, beginning at the base of the left trunk and ending at the base of the right.

The primary causes of all illnesses are the three poisons of delusion, desire, and hatred. Due to delusion we view everything as permanent; this generates desire when experiences are pleasant, and anger when experiences are unpleasant. These three poisons cause an imbalance of the three *nyes-pas.*

The secondary causes of illnesses are improper diet, improper conduct, seasonal factors, and the influences of evil spirits.

1. The other authors of this volume translate *nyes-pa* as "humor." Dr. Bradley prefers to use the Tibetan term because in her opinion the concept is in some ways different from the traditional Western notion of the humors of wind, bile, and phlegm, terms for which Dr. Bradley instead uses air, fire, and fluid, respectively.

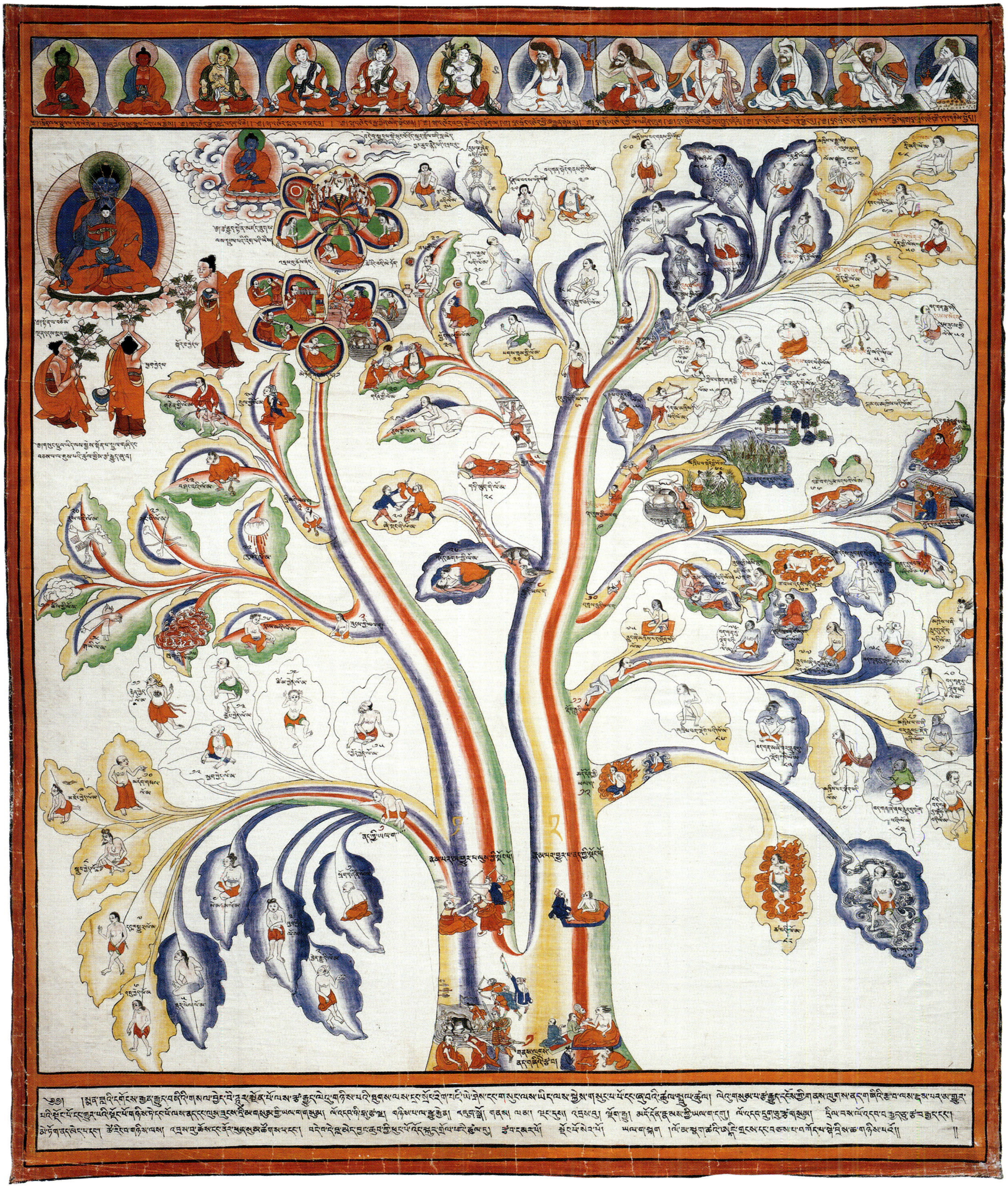

3. Human Embryology

This painting shows human conception, development, and childbirth.

Conception has primary and secondary causes. The primary causes are the father's semen, the mother's menstrual blood, and the consciousness that enters the womb, influenced by past-life karma, delusion, desire, and hatred. The semen and menstrual blood should both be healthy; the semen should be white in color, thick, plenty like honey, and sweet in taste, and the menstrual blood should be like red rabbit blood; if it stains it is easily washed. In Tibetan medicine there are nine defects relating to the semen and menstrual blood that may prevent conception. These are here illustrated by the first nine egglike forms.

In addition to the semen, menstrual blood, and consciousness, we need the five elements of earth, water, fire, air, and space; these are the secondary causes of conception. Earth helps the fetus to be solid; water helps it to cohere; fire to mature; air helps it to grow; and space helps it to move.

The father's semen generates bone, the brain, and the spinal cord, while the mother's menstrual blood generates muscle tissue, the five full organs, and the six hollow organs. Consciousness develops the five senses.

Earth generates muscle tissue, bone, and the nose and its sense of smell. Water generates blood, bodily fluids, and the tongue and its sense of taste. Fire generates heat, clarity of complexion, and the eyes and their sense of sight. Air generates breath, as well as the skin and its sense of touch. Space generates various orifices, among them the ears and their sense of hearing.

The embryo is thus formed by having healthy semen and menstrual blood, consciousness, and the five elements.

The behavior and diet of the mother are very important for healthy development. She should avoid strenuous physical exertion, late nights, sleeping in the daytime, and eating hot and sharp foods. She should have plenty of fiber; inappropriate diet and behavior may result in miscarriage or stillbirth.

Whatever the mother eats or drinks is digested by her digestive system, and its essence is stored in her reproductive organs. They are connected to the two channels of the uterus by the umbilical cord, which in turn develops the fetus.

The development of the fetus takes thirty-eight weeks. In the fish stage of development (weeks one through nine) the fetus is fish-shaped, with no visible limbs. In the turtle stage (weeks ten through seventeen) the fetus is turtle-shaped; the limbs have appeared, as have the five full organs, the six hollow organs, the sense organs, and the connective nerves and channels. In the pig stage (weeks eighteen through thirty-five) everything is developed and functional; it is called the pig stage because the fetus can now feel the dirtiness of its surroundings.

After thirty-eight weeks the fetus turns upside down and is ready for delivery. Symptoms are heavy feelings in the lower body, excruciating back pains, expansion of the vagina, and the frequent passing of urine. It is then important to properly care for the mother and child after birth.

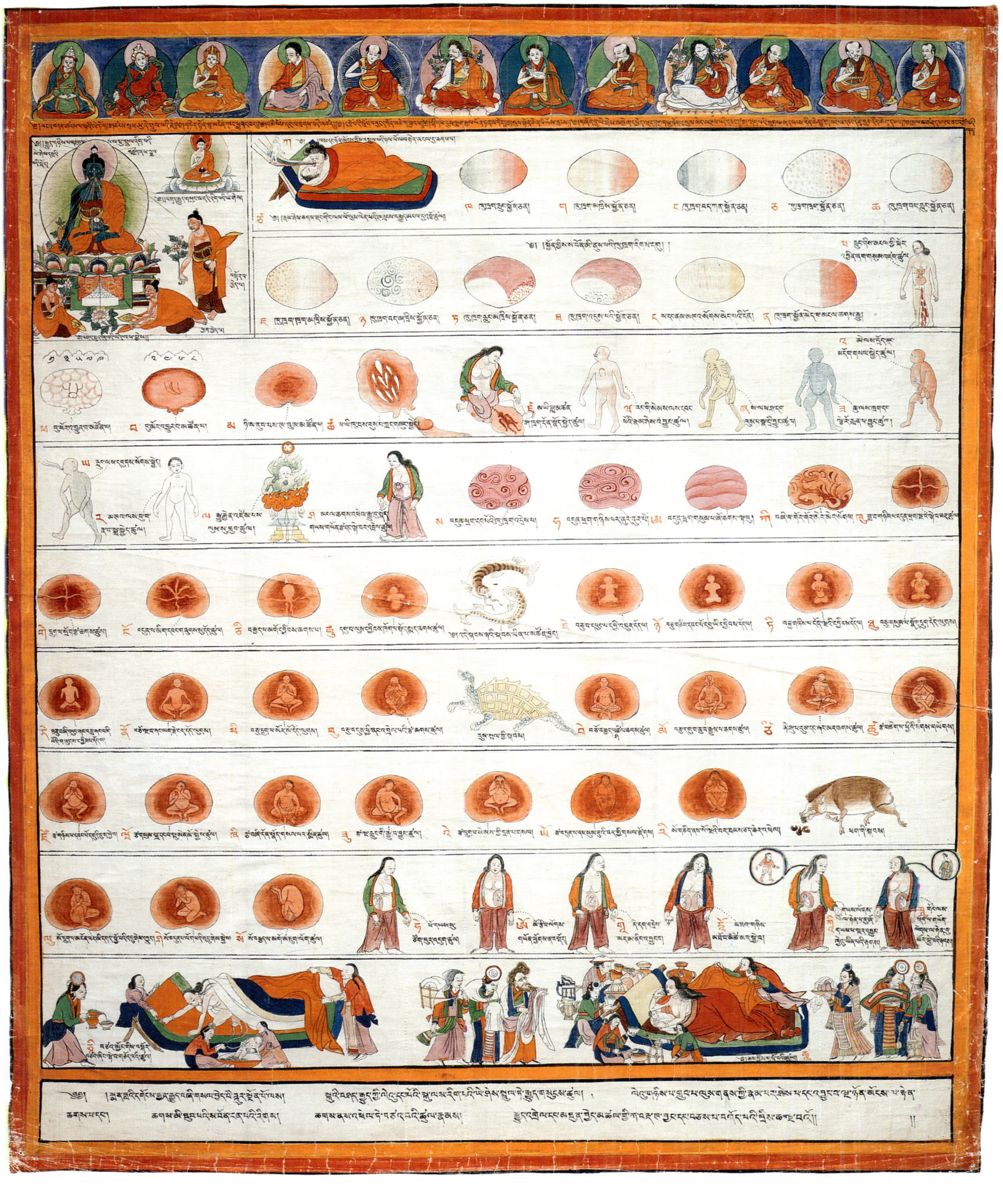

4. *Metaphors and Measurements of the Body*

This painting shows metaphors and measurements of the human body. Its purpose is to provide a lay person with an understanding of physical anatomy.

To describe the physical body, visualize a person sitting cross-legged with a straight back, arms resting gently on the knees. This figure is like the palace of a universal emperor.

The hip bones are like the walls of the palace foundations, the vertebrae like a stack of gold coins, the ribs like the palace beams, the flesh and skin like the plaster of the building, the head like a palace turret, the five sense organs like the palace windows, and the upper and lower parts of the trunk like the upper and lower courtyards of the palace.

The five full organs—heart, lungs, liver, spleen, and kidneys—can be compared as follows. In the upper courtyard the heart is like a king sitting on a throne, the lungs are like ministers of the king, the liver and spleen are like the senior and junior queens, and the kidneys are like the king's foreign ministers.

The six hollow organs—stomach, intestine, large intestine, gall bladder, urinary bladder, and reproductive organs—can be compared as follows. The stomach is like a cooking pot, the intestine and large intestine are like the queen's housemaids, the gall bladder is like a sack full of spices, the urinary bladder is like a water jar, and the two lower passages of the anus and urethra are like two drainage gutters.

Finally, the legs are like arch pediments above the palace gates.

Tibetan medicine is over 2,500 years old. As it naturally was without a metric system, the volume measurements in this picture are in the form of a single handful and a cupped handful. The traditional forms of measurement are based on a healthy adult man.

The right quantity of *rlung* is equal to the volume of the urinary bladder, the right quantity of *mkhris-pa* is equal to the capacity of the scrotum, and the right quantity of *bad-kan* is equal to three cupped handfuls.

The amount of blood and feces in the body should be equal to seven cupped handfuls, urine should be equal to four cupped handfuls, the brain equal to one cupped handful, and semen equal to one single handful.

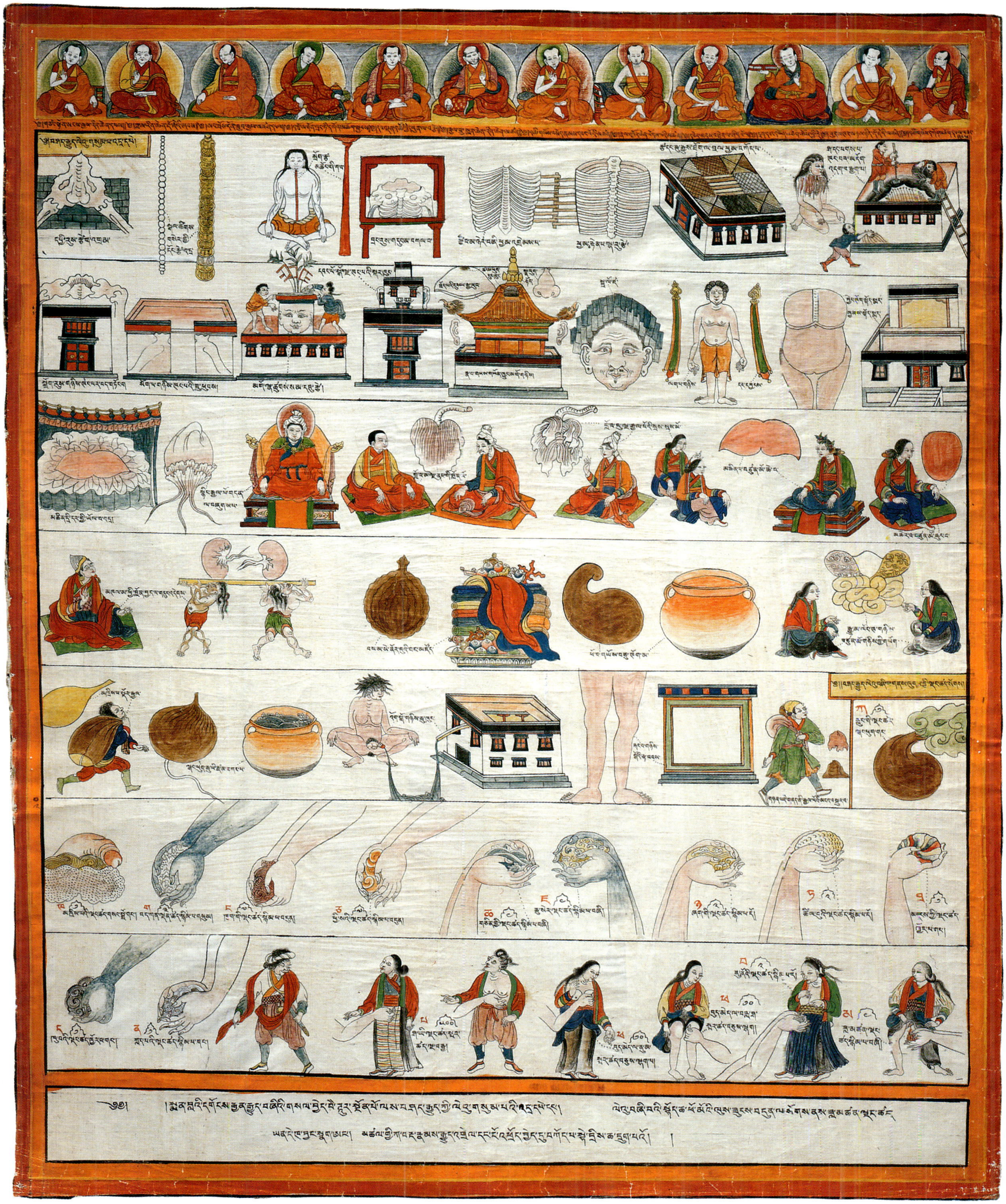

5. *Anatomy: Front View*

This painting shows the anterior view of the human anatomy. In the painting, bones are classified into twenty-three different groupings.

For the cranial bones there are five groups: the skull, occipital bones, nasal bones, teeth, and mandible.

For the trunk there are nine groups: vertebrae, sacrum, coccyx, hip bones, shoulder bones, collar bones, sternum, ribs, and costal cartilages.

For the arms there are three groups: humerus; forearm, including the radius and ulna; and the hand, including carpals, metacarpals, and phalanges.

For the legs there are five groups: femur; lower leg, including tibia and fibula; patella; calcaneus; and the foot, including the tarsals, metatarsals, and phalanges.

Finally, there is a single group comprising the fingernails and toenails.

All the bones are connected by 12 major joints and 210 minor joints.

The human body is covered with thirty-five million pores, and on the head there are twenty-one thousand hairs.

Also shown in this painting are the five full organs (heart, lungs, liver, spleen, and kidneys), and the six hollow organs (stomach, small intestine, large intestine, gall bladder, urinary bladder, and reproductive organs).

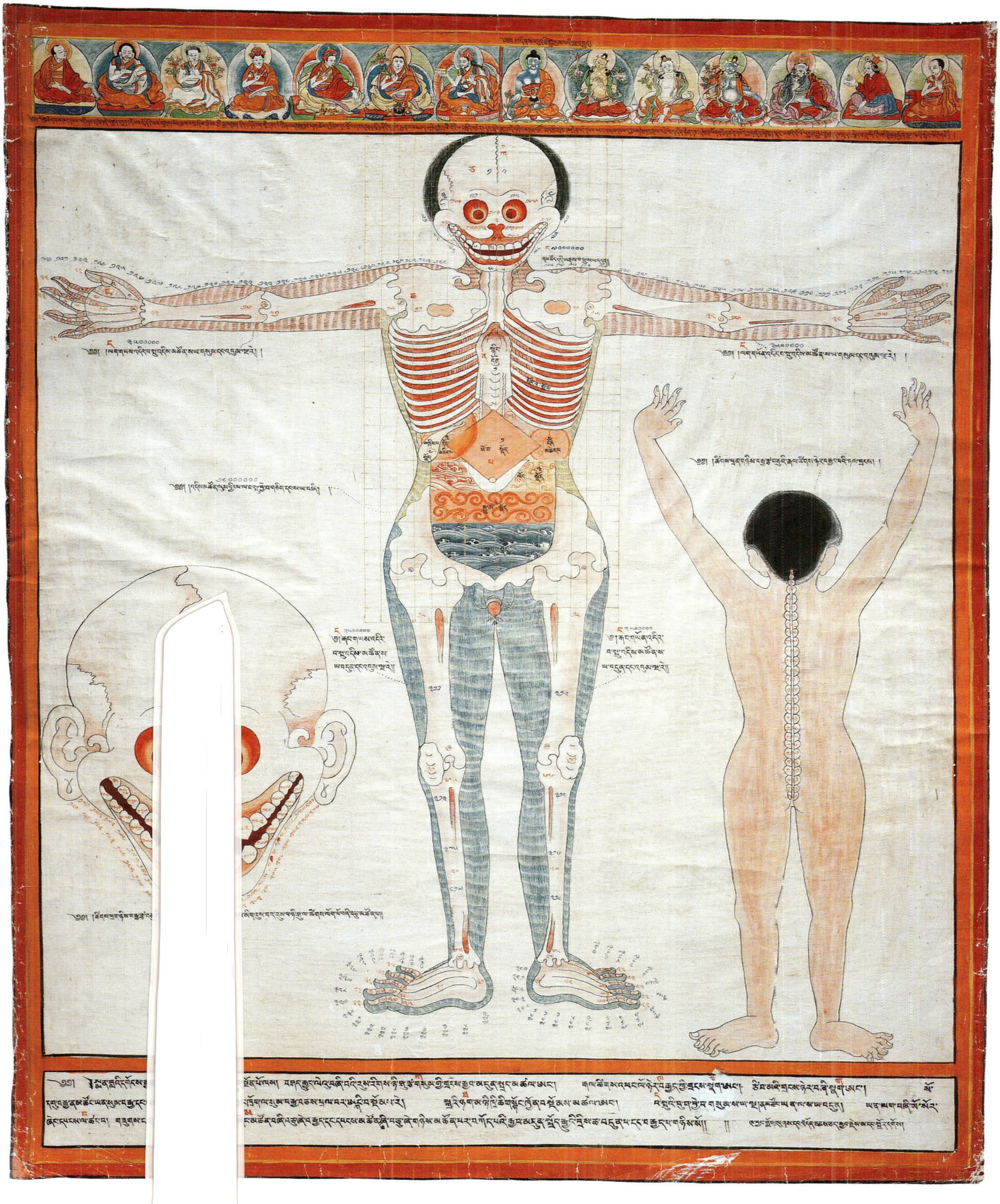

6. *Blood Vessels: Front View*

This painting shows the four different types of channels *(rtsa)* in Tibetan medicine: embryonic formation channels, existent channels, connecting channels, and lifespan channels. Where the channels intertwine, *chakras* are formed.

The embryonic formation channel extends from the navel and divides into three subchannels. The first subchannel extends upward to form the brain. The brain is the source of all our thoughts and also the source of our ignorance. It is the location of *bad-kan.* When we feel confused and heavy, the feeling begins in our head. The second subchannel is the hepatic artery of the liver, and it forms the black channel of life and blood vessels. Blood is the cause of the heat that generates anger. It is also the location of *mkhris-pa,* in the middle part of our body. The third subchannel extends down to form the genitalia, which are the source of pleasure. This channel generates desire, and is the location of *rlung,* in the lower part of the body.

The sensory organs are connected by five hundred minor existent channels to the brain. To enhance the memory, there are five hundred minor existent channels connected to the heart *chakra.* The human body originates from the five hundred minor channels in the navel *chakra.* Offspring originate in the genitalia *chakra.*

All the channels are connected to each other throughout the body like a net.

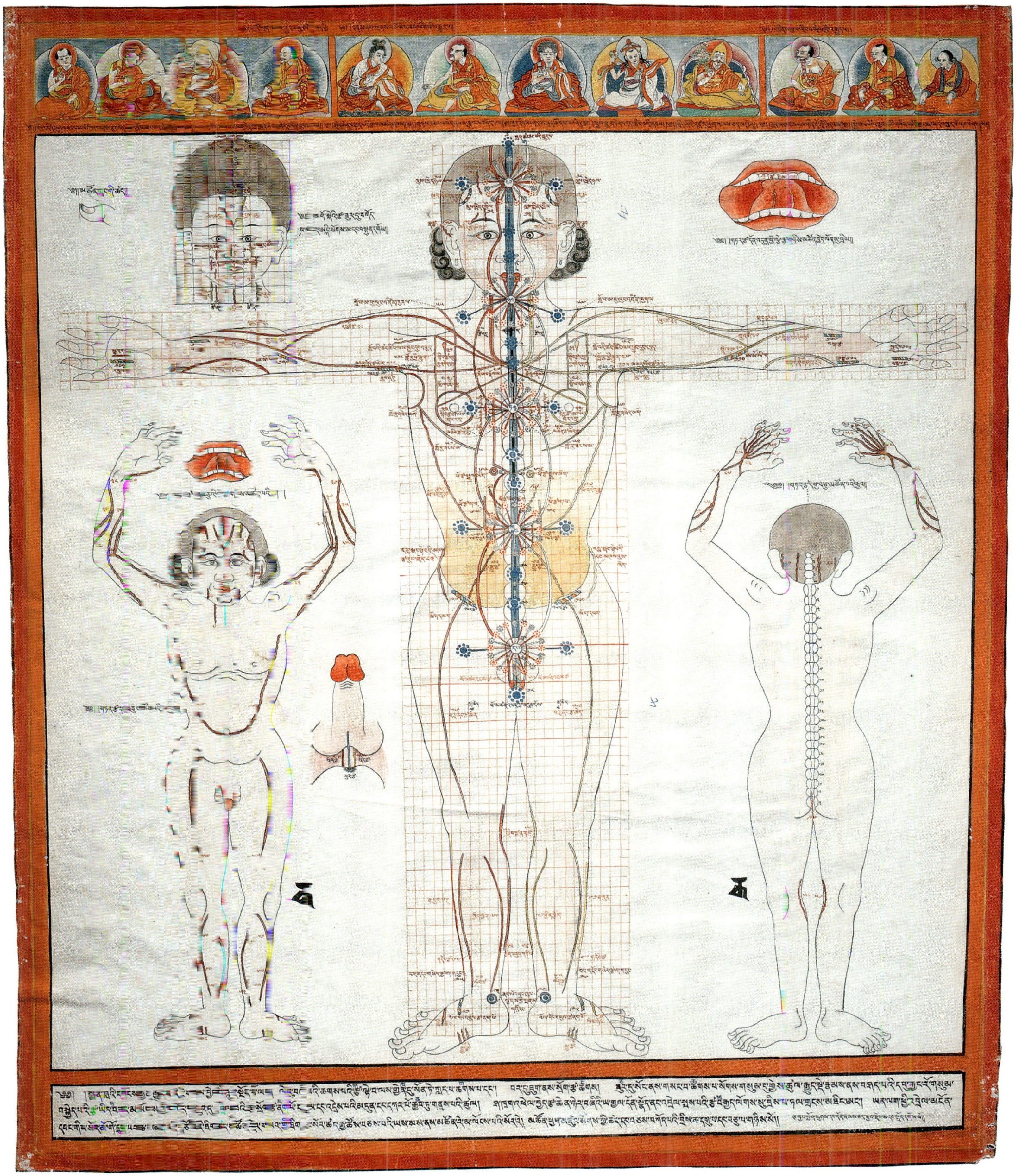

7. Blood Vessels: Back View

This is a continuation from the preceding painting, plate 6.

The connecting channels are divided into the black channel and the white channel. The black channel is called the life channel because it sustains life. Without blood we are unable to survive; thus the black channel originates from the liver, where the twenty-four major blood vessels also originate. It helps to sustain muscle tissue and blood. Eight of the twenty-four blood vessels are connected internally to the five full and six hollow organs, as seen in the left figure. The sixteen external blood vessels are connected to the limbs. There are 77 bloodletting vessels, and 112 vulnerable blood vessels that cannot be used for bloodletting as that would be fatal; in addition, there are 360 minor blood vessels. The figure on the right shows the heart *chakra (dharmachakra),* through which the consciousness of the senses flows.

In Tibetan medicine, one's lifespan depends on past karma, as well as one's diet and behavior in this life. The essence of reproductive fluid is called *dhang* or *ojas,* which flows throughout the body but is concentrated in the heart. It sustains life, and is responsible for bodily lustre. The lifespan channels are divided into three.

The first lifespan channel flows from head to toe in a thirty-day lunar cycle. In the male body, *bla* (life energy) flows from left to right, and in the female body it flows from right to left. The physician must know the exact whereabouts of the *bla* when performing therapies such as bloodletting and moxibustion. For example, on the first day of the lunar calendar the syllable *ah* is flowing in the big toe of the male patient, and therefore performing moxibustion on that point is not advisable.

The second lifespan channel circulates with the breath.

The third lifespan channel contains the *bla* that can be felt by the physician at the edge of the wrist. This energy sometimes disappears, escaping through the ring finger to wander externally. During that time a lama or advanced tantric practitioner can perform long-life prayers for the patient, in an attempt to recapture the wandering *bla.* In Tibetan society, if it was said that someone's *bla* had gone, it meant they would soon die. Their face would appear as if drained of all life.

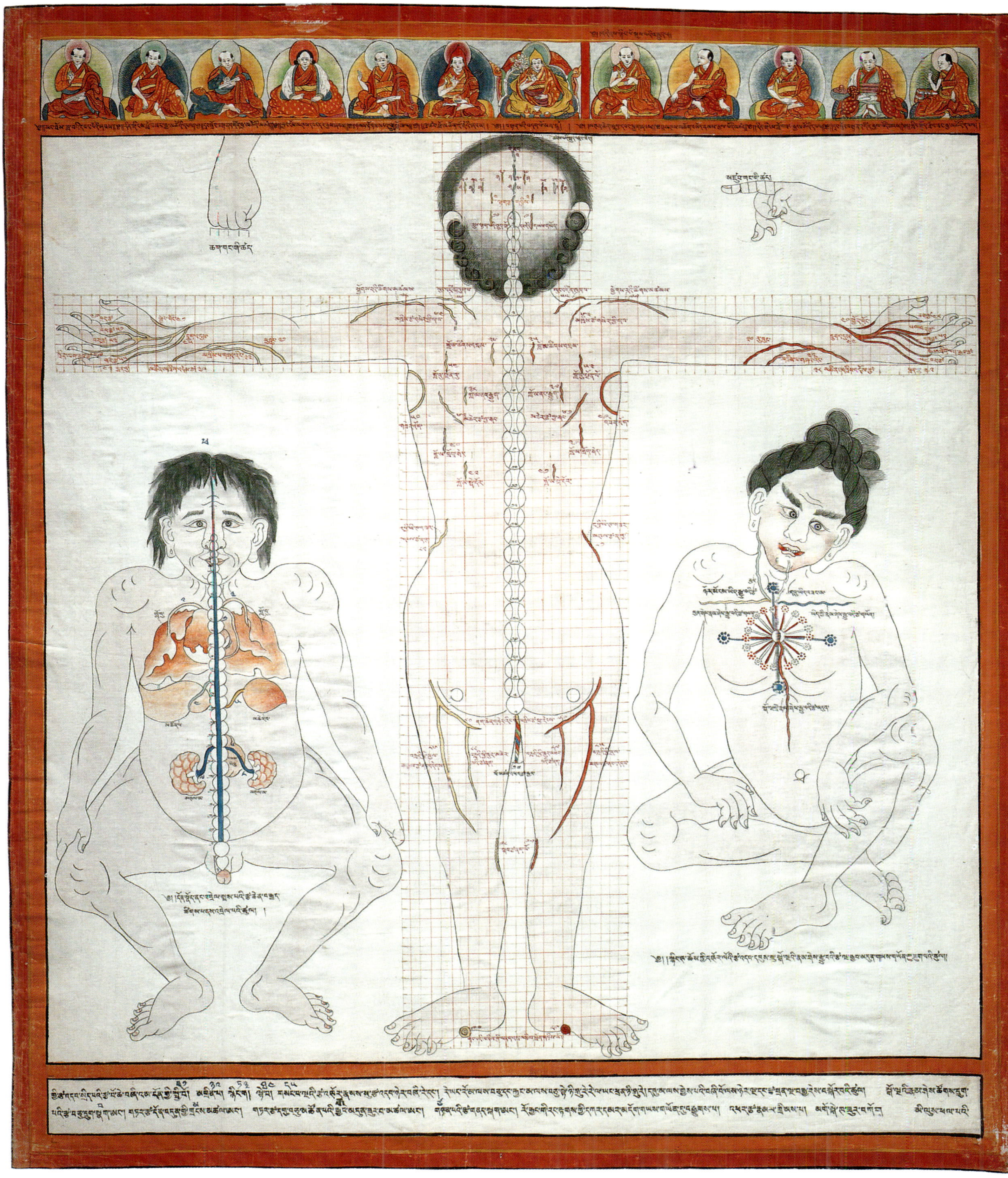

8. *White Channels: The Nervous System*

The preceding painting (plate 7) described the black channel. This painting shows the white channel of life, consisting of the spinal cord and its connected nerves. Its stem is located in the brain; the channel runs down through the vertebrae and ends at the coccyx. The main function of the white channel is to regulate the water element (cerebrospinal fluid) throughout the body.

There are roughly nineteen major white channels. Four are connected to the heart and small intestines, and they help the functioning of *rlung.* Four are connected to the lungs, large intestines, liver, and gall bladder, and they help the functioning of *mkhris-pa.* Four are connected with the stomach, spleen, kidneys, and urinary bladder, and they help the functioning of *bad-kan.* There is one common white channel connected to the reproductive organs. There are six external white channels: two tubular, two precious, and two paralytic channels. The tubular channels are more hollow than normal channels, the precious channels are life-sustaining, and the paralytic channels are so named due to the fact that if they are injured, a person can become paralyzed.

In addition, there are eleven minor white channels.

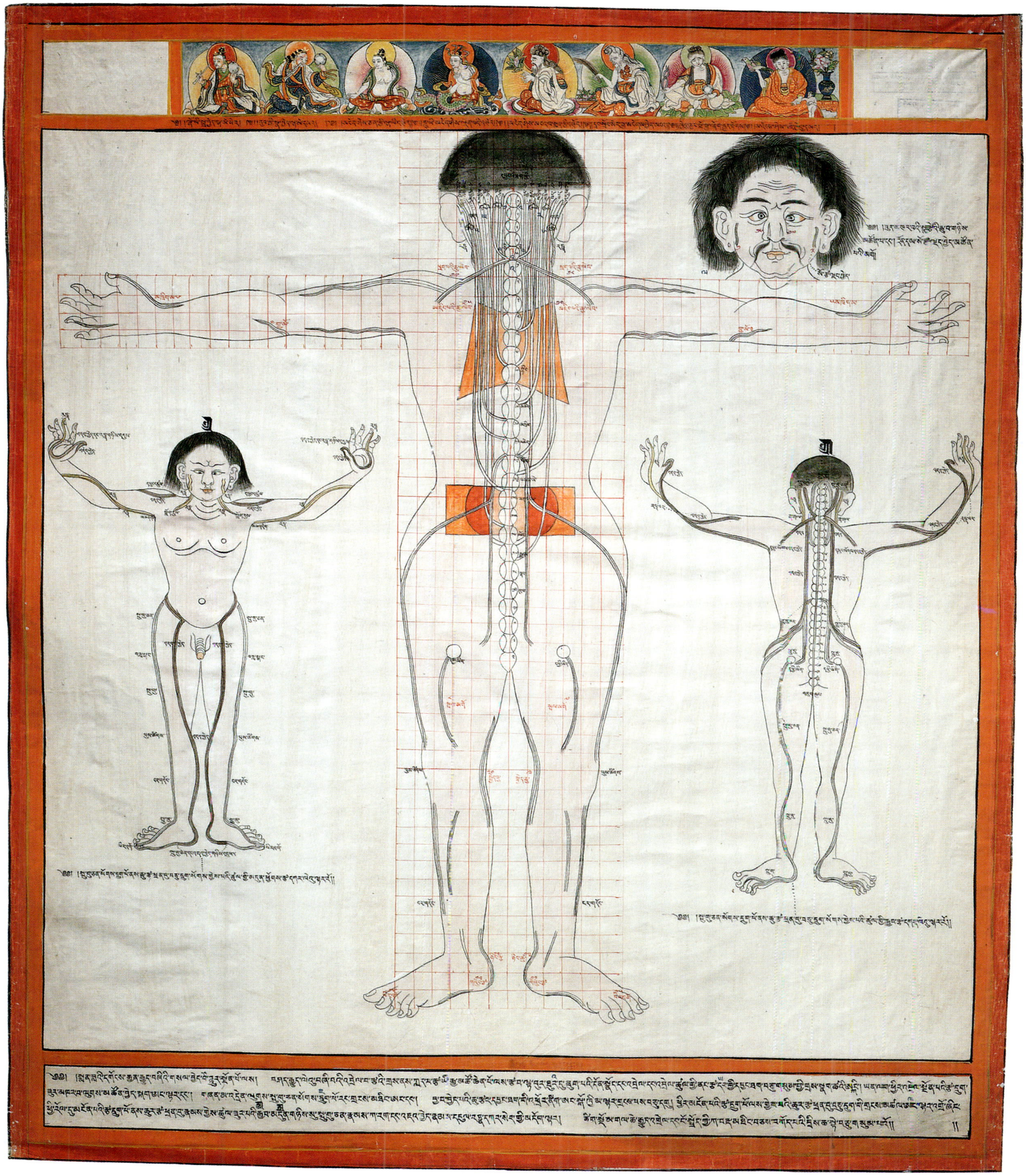

9. The Organs

This painting shows the exact location of the five full organs and six hollow organs. It is very important for the physician to know the exact location of the organs in order to perform external therapies such as bloodletting and moxibustion. If the exact locations of these organs are not known, these therapies will be inaccurate.

When checking the exact location of the organs the physician places the patient on a flat mattress. The patient sits cross-legged with a straight back, head bent slightly forward, shoulders pushed back, hands resting on the knees.

The upper and lower parts of the trunk are separated by the diaphragm.

The upper trunk consists of the lungs and heart. In Tibetan medical anatomy the lungs are divided into the five posterior lobes and the five anterior lobes. The posterior lobes are known in Tibetan as the "mother lungs" and they are situated at the back. The anterior lobes are known as the "son lungs" and they are situated in the front. The heart sits on top of the posterior lobes like a king on his throne.

The lower trunk (below the diaphragm) contains the remaining three full organs. The liver (on the right side) is compared to a rock sitting on a precipice and pointing upward. The spleen is thinner in the middle and thicker at the outer edges, and it is located just below the stomach. The left and right kidneys are in an upright position, and are compared to bodyguards.

Of the six hollow organs the stomach is the storage space for ingested food; its shape is wider in the upper part and narrower in the lower part. The small intestine, connected to the stomach, is like a gutter filled with water. The large intestine is connected to the small intestine and it is divided into three sections: the ascending, transverse, and descending colons. The sigmoid colon (flexure) and the rectum are connected to the large intestine. The gall bladder is connected to the liver and looks like a yellow pouch. The urinary bladder is like a storage jar, and the reproductive organs are like glands.

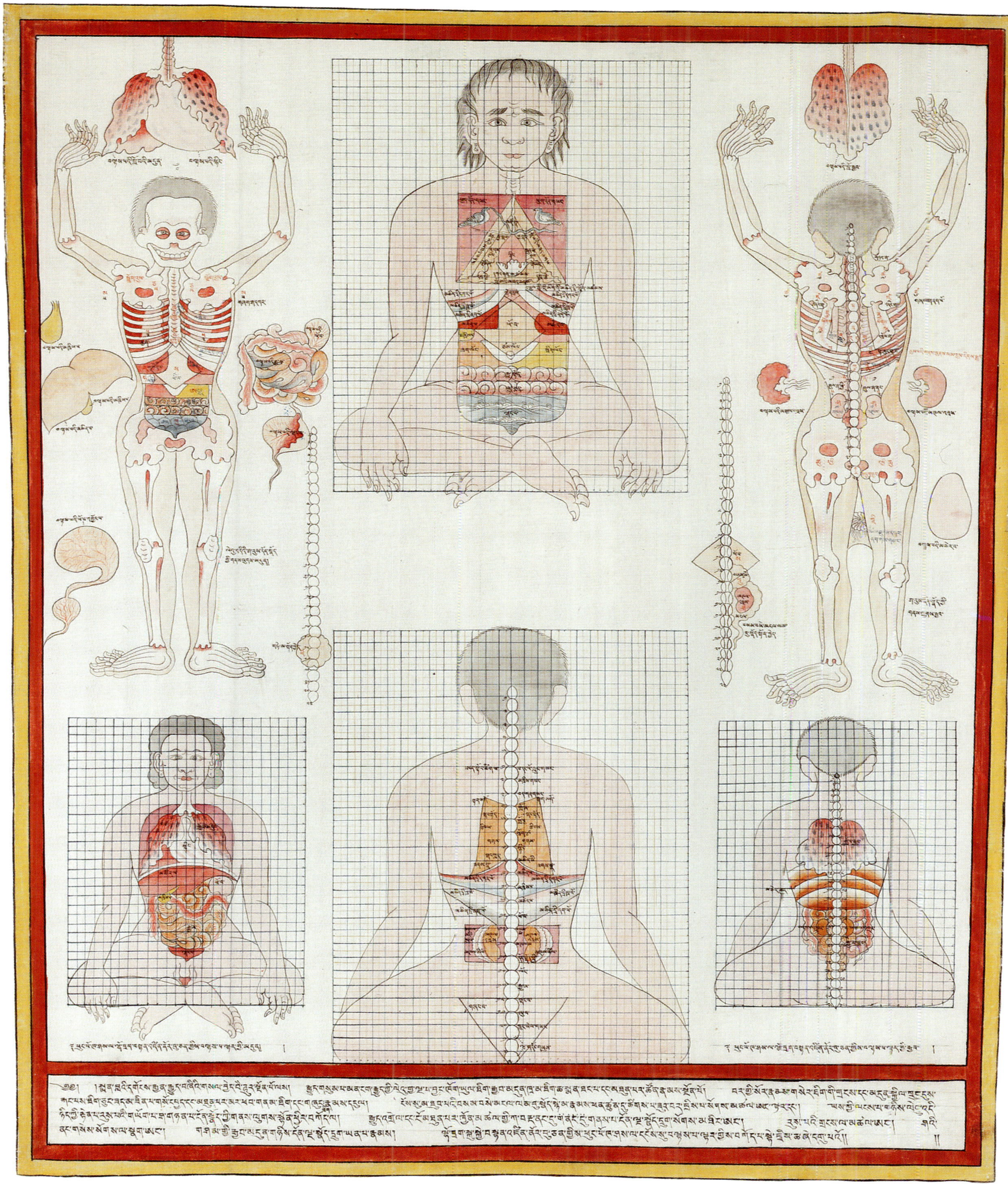

10. The Vulnerable Points of the Body: Front View

This painting shows the vulnerable points of the body. In Tibetan medicine they are divided into seven groups: points in the muscle tissue, fatty tissue, bones, ligaments, and tendons (shown in the center figure); full and hollow organs (shown in the left figure); and the channels (shown in the right figure).

They are vulnerable when struck and damaged by weapons. Muscle tissue swells up; if a bone is cracked or fractured there is unbearable pain; if the ligaments or tendons are damaged there is paralysis; if the channels, fatty tissue, or the full and hollow organs are damaged it is life-threatening.

There are a total of 322 vulnerable points in the body.

For muscle tissue there are five vulnerable points in the head, four in the neck, eighteen in the trunk, and eighteen in the limbs.

For fatty tissue there are two vulnerable points in the trunk and six in the limbs.

For bone tissue there are fourteen vulnerable points on the head, five in the neck, seven in the trunk, and six in the limbs.

For ligaments and tendons there are two vulnerable points in the neck, two in the trunk, and ten in the limbs.

For the full and hollow organs there are thirteen vulnerable points in the heart, lungs, liver, spleen, kidneys, stomach, gall bladder, small intestine, large intestine, urinary bladder, and reproductive organs.

For the channels there are fifteen vulnerable points in the brain, fourteen in the bone channels, fourteen in the muscle tissue, twenty-two in the neck, fifty-three in the trunk, and seventy-two in the limbs.

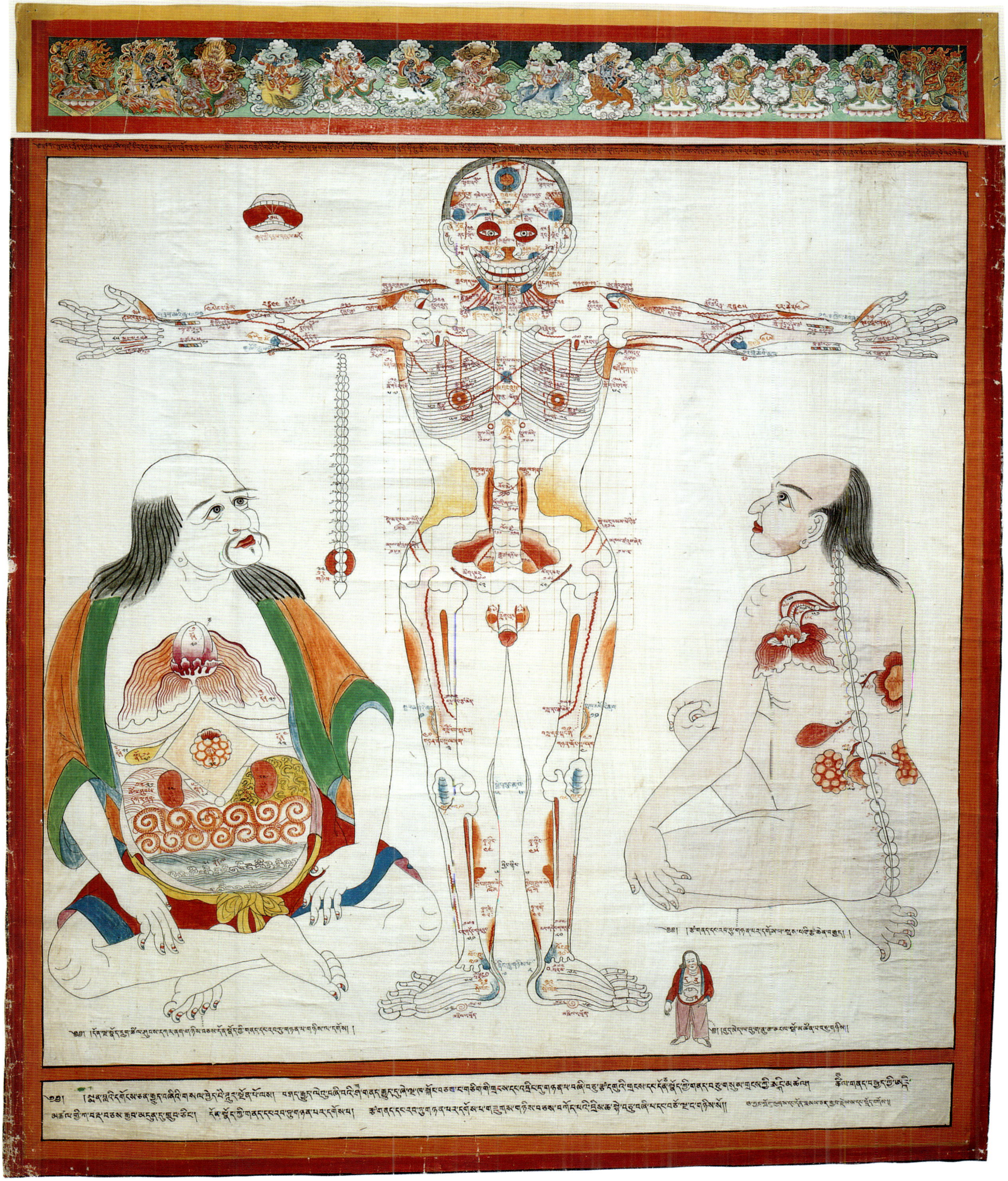

11. *The Three Nyes-pas*

This painting shows the different human genders, ages, and personality types. In Tibetan medical science, gender is divided into male, female, and hermaphrodite (shown on the far right of the second row). Age is also divided into three: ages one to sixteen are children, ages sixteen to seventy are adults, and those over seventy are aged. There are seven human types: *rlung, mkhris-pa,* and *bad-kan,* combinations of two of these together *(rlung/mkhris-pa, rlung/bad-kan, mkhris-pa/bad-kan),* and finally a combination of all three.

Of the three poisons of delusion, hatred, and desire, *rlung* people are most closely associated with desire. This is symbolized by a bird, which is seen as a very sexually active creature. *Rlung* people (shown beginning on the right side of the third row) are stout, stooping, thin, with a dark complexion, talkative, argumentative, and unable to bear the cold. They love songs and hunting, and they laugh easily. They will mostly suffer from anxiety and insomnia. They prefer foods that are sweet, sour, bitter, and hot. They will not be wealthy, and they will have a short lifespan. They are similar to vultures, crows, and foxes.

Mkhris-pa people are most closely associated with hatred. This is symbolized by a snake, which is seen as a very aggressive creature. *Mkhris-pa* people are intelligent, proud, and hot-tempered. Their complexion and hair are fair, they perspire easily, and they frequently feel hungry and thirsty. They prefer sweet, bitter, and astringent foods. Their wealth, lifespan, and height are all average. They are similar to monkeys, tigers, and *yakshas* (divine trickster spirits, often associated with the forest, that disturb the meditation of monks by making loud noises).

Bad-kan people are most closely associated with delusion. This is symbolized by the pig, which is seen as a very ignorant animal. Their body temperature is cold. They are of large build, with fair complexions. They are heavy sleepers, and they are very patient and kind. They are able to withstand thirst and hunger, like hot, sour, and astringent foods, will enjoy wealth and longevity, and are similar to lions, elephants, and eagles.

For a *rlung* and *mkhris-pa* combination the person will be a combination of the *rlung* and *mkhris-pa* characteristics. This also applies to all the other combinations that make up the seven personality types.

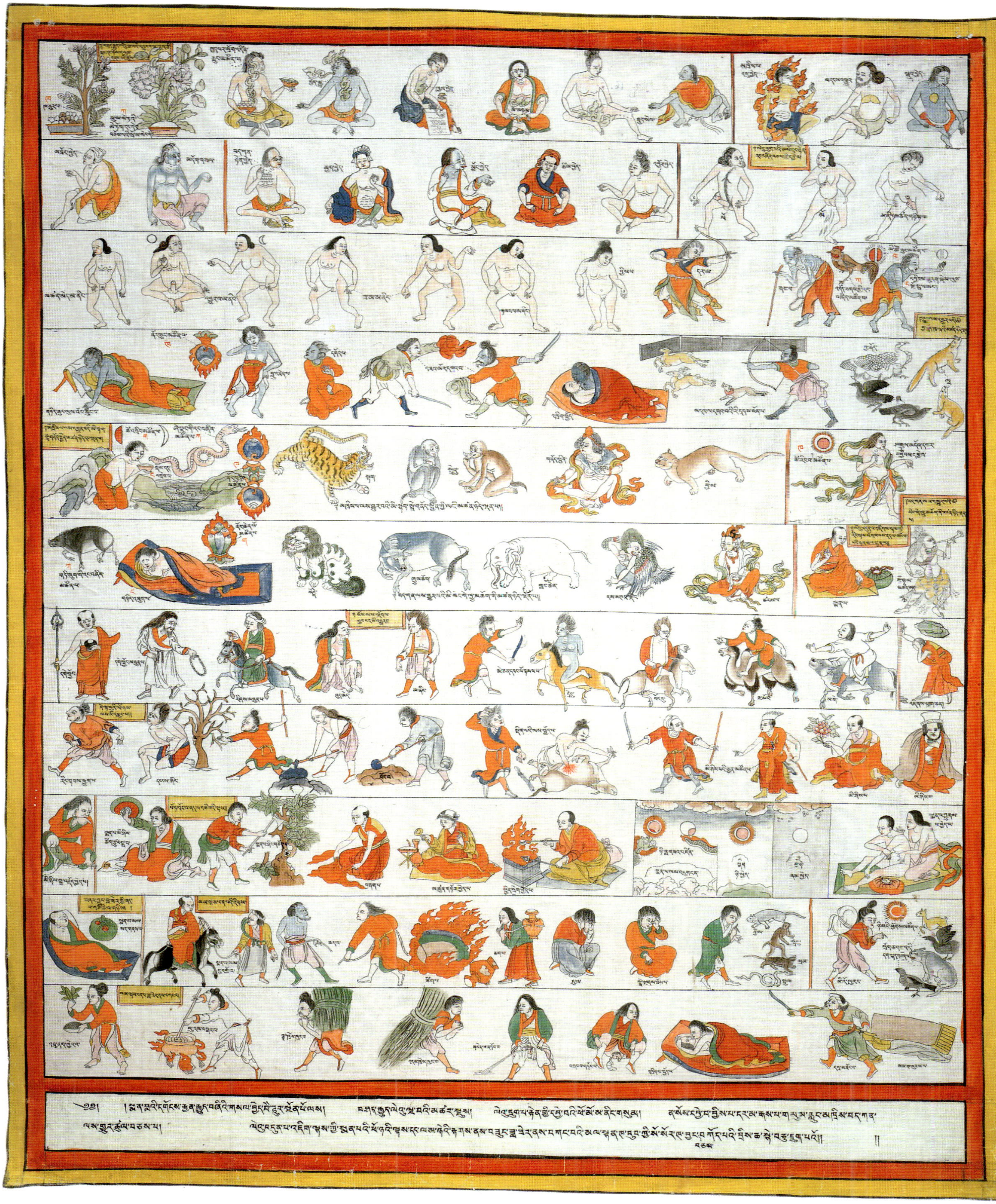

12. *Humoral Disorders and their Causes*

The primary causes of disease are illustrated in the top register: ignorance (which is the general, fundamental cause), desire, hatred, and delusion.

The theory of Tibetan medicine is to keep in balance the three *nyes-pas* of *rlung, mkhris-pa,* and *bad-kan;* the seven bodily constituents; and the three excretory functions. If there is an excess or deficiency of these in our body, or if they are aggravated, it can lead to illness.

Of the three *nyes-pas,* when *mkhris-pa* is in excess, feces, urine, skin, and sclera turn yellow; the patient becomes excessively hungry and thirsty, feverish, is unable to sleep, and has diarrhea. When there is a deficiency of *mkhris-pa,* the body temperature is low, and the patient's complexion darkens. When *mkhris-pa* is aggravated, the pulse is fast, overflowing, and taut; the urine is reddish yellow and has a strong odor and vapor. The patient will have headaches, a bitter taste in the mouth, a thick coating on the tongue, sleepiness in the daytime, excess of thirst, diarrhea with a strong odor and sometimes with bleeding, and post-digestive pain at midday and midnight.

Of the seven bodily constituents, when there is excess muscle tissue there is the appearance of goiter, swollen glands, and an increase in weight. When there is a deficiency in muscle tissue there is loss of weight, and pain in the joints—as if there were no tissue to hold them together.

Of the three excretory functions, an excess of feces will result in heaviness in the body, flatulence, rumbling in the stomach, pain in the intestines, and the patient will not feel like moving. A deficiency of feces will result in a throbbing pain in the ribs due to wind in the intestine, and pain in the heart.

When the three *nyes-pas* are imbalanced it can affect the functioning of the seven bodily constituents, the three excretory functions, the five senses, the five full organs, and the six hollow organs. When *rlung* is located in the bones and joints, it causes ringing in the ears, the skin becomes dry and rough, and there is pain in the large intestine. When *mkhris-pa* is located in the stomach it affects the blood, serum, eyes, and the small intestine. When *bad-kan* is located in the chest it affects the throat, lungs, head, fatty tissues, marrow, generative fluid, feces, and urine, and it especially affects the nose and the tongue.

In Tibetan medicine there are 404 diseases, which can be placed into four main categories: 101 untreatable diseases caused by past karma; 101 diseases caused by spirits, which can be eliminated through rituals; 101 diseases caused by improper diet and improper behavior in this life, which can be cured by medication; and 101 ostensible diseases causing minor injuries and illnesses, which can be cured easily, without the help of medication.

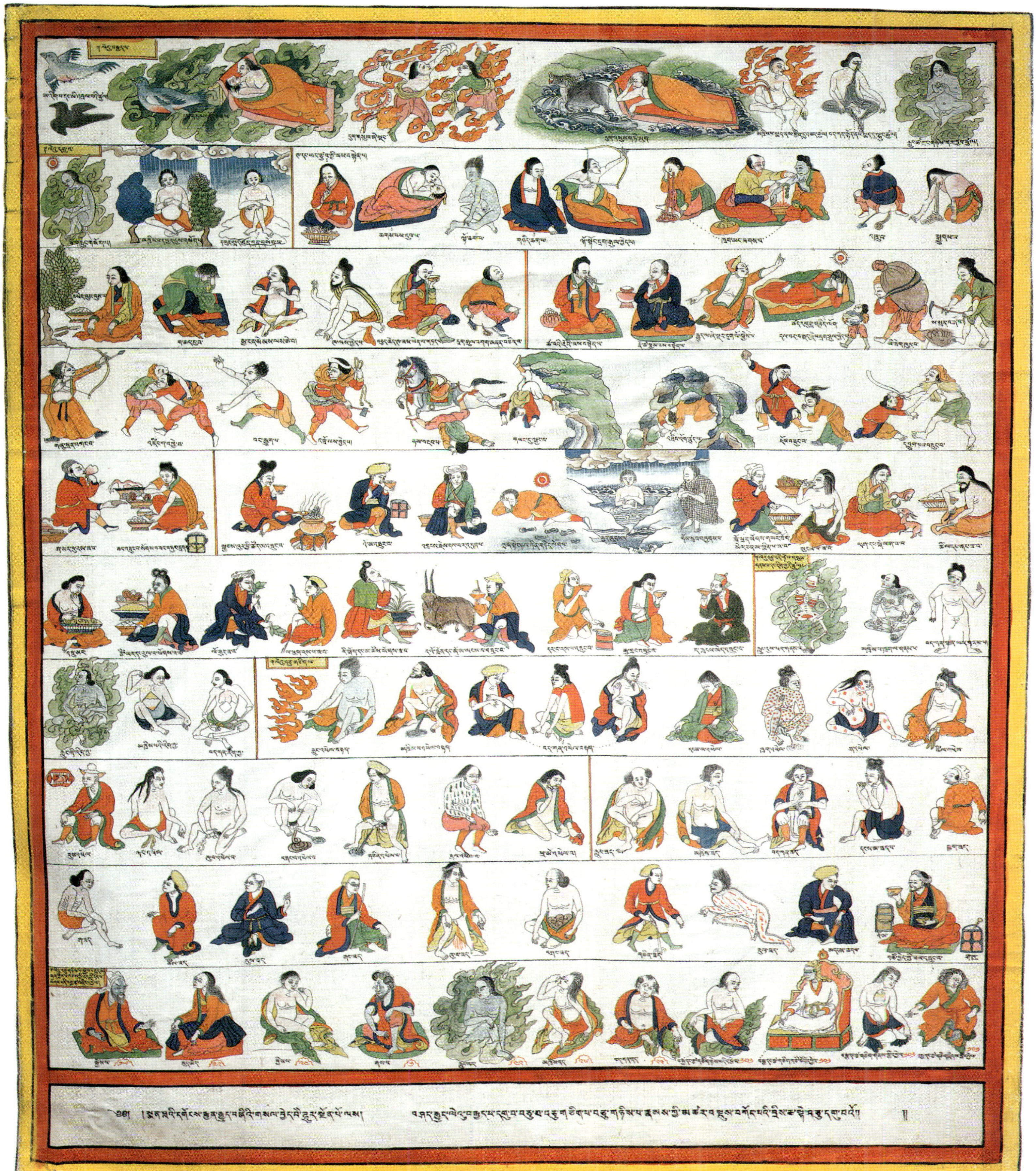

13. *The Tree of Diagnosis*

In this painting the blue leaves symbolize *rlung,* the yellow leaves *mkhris-pa,* and the white leaves *bad-kan.*

This painting shows how Tibetan physicians diagnose illness when the three *nyes-pas* are imbalanced.

The root of diagnosis has three trunks: visual observation, pulse reading, and questioning.

Visual observation (the left trunk) consists of checking the tongue, and uroscopy. The tongue of a *rlung* patient is reddish with a coarse, dry texture. The *mkhris-pa* patient's tongue is covered with a thick yellowish coating. The *bad-kan* patient's tongue is white, pale, smooth, and wet.

The urine of a *rlung* patient is like water when stirred, with big bubbles; the *mkhris-pa* patient's urine is reddish yellow, with a strong odor and thick vapor; the *bad-kan* patient's urine is white, with very little odor and vapor.

Pulse reading (the middle trunk): The *rlung* patient's pulse is floating, empty when pressed, and is irregular. The *mkhris-pa* patient's pulse is fast, overflowing, and taut. The *bad-kan* patient's pulse is sunken, weak, and slow.

Questioning (the right trunk): The physician must ask questions about the symptoms of the illness, the location of the pain, and which foods harm or help the patient.

Rlung imbalance is aggravated by an excessive intake of light and rough food such as pork, goat meat, or strong tea or coffee; and by conduct such as fasting or exposure to cold winds. Symptoms indicative of *rlung* imbalance are yawning, frequent sighing, cold chills, pain in the bones and joints, anxiety, shifting pains, and dullness of the senses. Imbalance is confirmed if these symptoms are alleviated by eating oily, nutritious foods, and by leading a quiet lifestyle.

Mkhris-pa imbalance is aggravated by an excessive intake of heat-producing foods such as alcohol, lamb, butter, or oily foods; and conduct such as exposure to the sun and doing strenuous physical work. Symptoms indicative of *mkhris-pa* imbalance are headaches, a bitter taste in the mouth, fever, nausea, and post-digestive pain. Imbalance is confirmed when the symptoms are alleviated by eating foods and drinks with a cooling potency such as vegetables, mountain water, and nongreasy and low-fat foods.

Bad-kan imbalance is aggravated by exposure to cold; a heavy diet of foods such as full-fat milk and cheese, salads, and cold food; and by doing little exercise. Symptoms indicative of *bad-kan* imbalance are a loss of appetite, indigestion, excessive flatulence, and feeling cold and tired. Imbalance is confirmed when the symptoms are alleviated by eating warm, cooked foods, and by exercising.

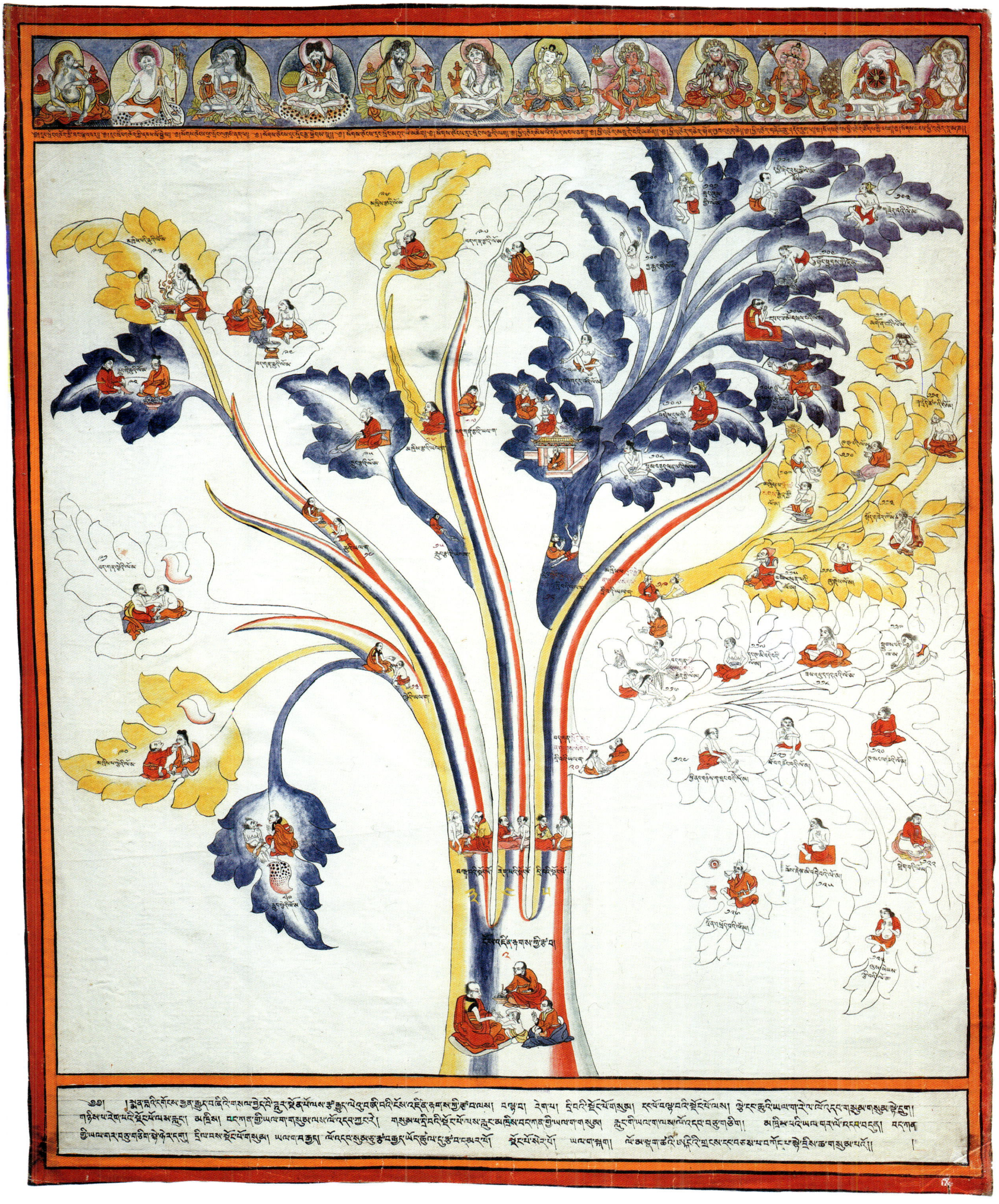

14. Dreams and Omens Revealing the Outcome of Disease

Within the Tibetan Buddhist cycle of life there is birth, aging and disease, and death.

Tibetan medical science is able to detect impending death through various signs of physical decay, which can be divided into four categories: long-term signs of decay, short-term signs of decay, uncertain signs, and certain signs.

Long-term signs of decay can be observed through dreams, behavior, and messengers (in Tibet if a patient was too ill to see a doctor in person, a messenger would be sent instead). If a patient dreams they are riding naked on a buffalo, horse, pig, donkey, or camel, and traveling in a southerly direction, it is a sign of decay. If a patient's behavior changes dramatically from calm to violent, and they suddenly begin to criticize their physician, their spiritual teacher, and they refuse to take any medicine, it is also a sign of decay. If the messenger is in a panic when he reaches the doctor, looks nervous, and arrives on a date that is astrologically inauspicious, it is also a sign of the decay of the patient.

Short-term signs of decay can be observed in connection with the five elements of earth, water, fire, air, and space—and the dissolution of these elements in the human body. Earth is absorbed by water and vision becomes blurred; water is absorbed by fire and causes the bodily cavities to dry up; fire is absorbed by air and there is loss of body heat; and air is absorbed by space and breathing ceases.

Short-term signs of decay are also observed in diminishing powers of the five sensory organs, seen in various external physical signs. When the sense of sight diminishes, vision becomes blurred and the eyes roll upward. When hearing diminishes, the patient is unable to hear anything and the ears become cupped. When smell diminishes, the patient is unable to smell anything and the nostrils become distended. When taste diminishes, the patient is unable to taste anything and there is a loss of voice, the tongue becomes dry and black in the middle, the lower lip hangs down, and the upper lip rolls upward. Finally, when the sense of touch diminishes, the patient is unable to feel anything.

From the Tibetan Buddhist perspective this is now a crucial moment for deciding the patient's future rebirth. Therefore it is very important that the patient has a calm mind. In Tibet, to ensure that the patient dies as peacefully as possible, spiritual practices, such as reciting Buddhist scriptures—for example, the *Bardo thödol*—are performed.

Uncertain signs of death include inauspicious dreams during illness. However, when the illness ceases, so do the dreams.

Certain signs of death include: when the patient is unable to take food; or when there are only bones and no muscle tissue, no pulse, and no response to any form of treatment.

It is vital for a qualified physician to be able to detect and predict impending death in order to preserve his good reputation.

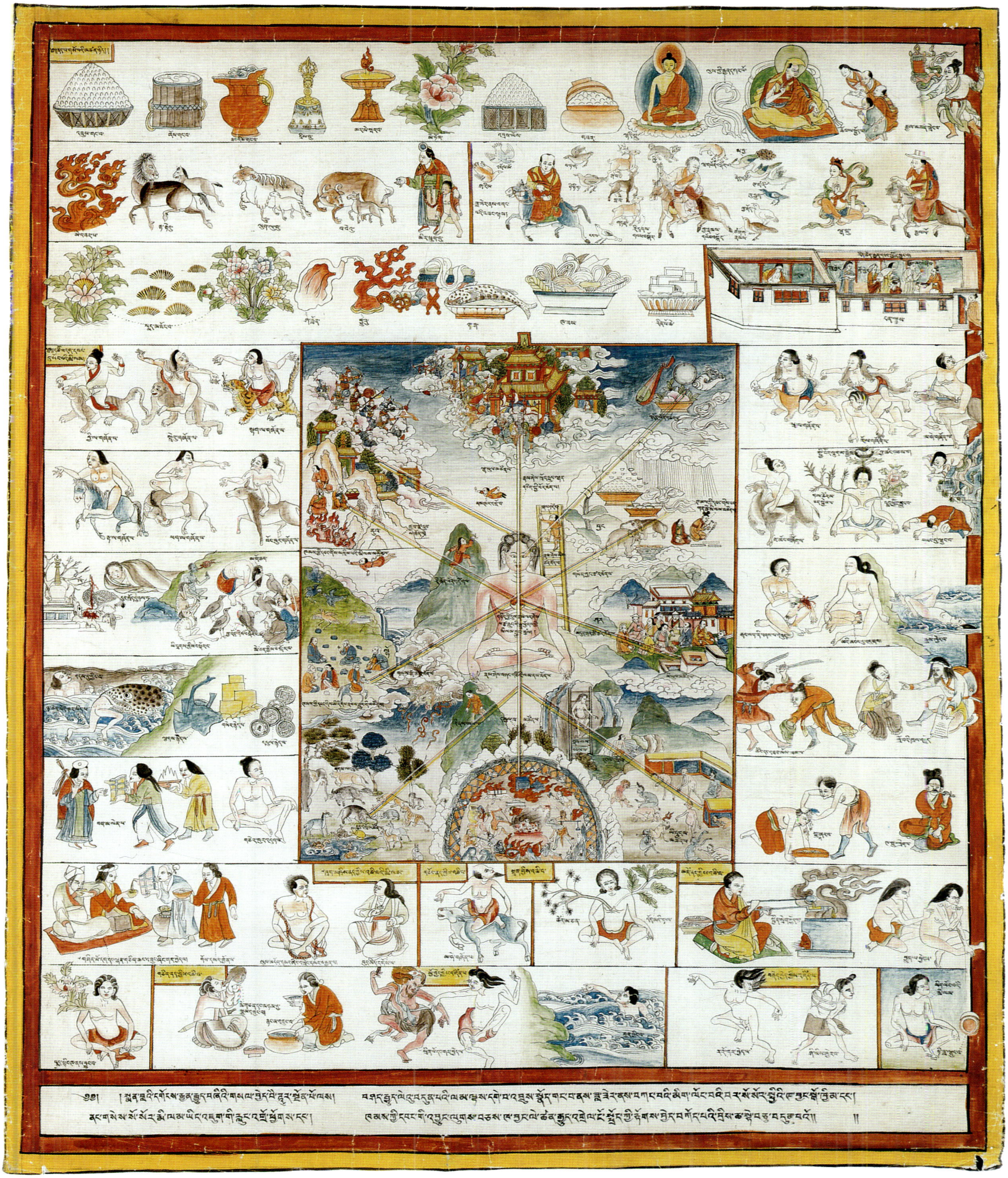

15. Feeling the Pulse: Diagnosis and Divination

This painting is divided into thirteen sections: 1. advice on diet and behavior the night before a pulse reading; 2. proper time for reading the pulse; 3. location of pulse reading; 4. pressure to be placed when reading the pulse; 5. how to read the pulse; 6. three constitutional pulses; 7. seasonal pulses; 8. seven wonder pulses; 9. differences between healthy and diseased pulses; 10. pulses indicative of disease; 11. death pulse; 12. demonic pulse; and 13. lifespan pulse.

The night before having one's pulse read, one should avoid meat, alcohol, heavy food, overeating or having an empty stomach, sexual intercourse, staying up late, excessive talking, and too much mental activity.

In the human body there are three main subtle channels: *rKyang-ma, Roma,* and *dBu-ma.* The *rKyang-ma* channel is influenced by the moon, *Roma* by the sun, and *dBu-ma* by neutral energy. At night the pulse is slower because the lunar influence is stronger, and in the daytime the solar influence is stronger and the pulse is faster and stronger. At dawn, when the lines on the palms are visible, these influences are in a dynamic state of equilibrium, and therefore that is the best time to read the pulse.

The place to read the pulse is the radial artery at the first crease of the wrist. The physician uses his index, middle, and ring fingers. The index finger is pressed lightly to feel the skin, the middle is pressed with medium pressure to feel the muscle tissue, and the ring finger is pressed hard to feel the bone.

For pulse reading the fingers of the physician should be supple and of the right temperature. If the patient is male the physician's right hand reads the left arm of the patient. The index finger reads the heart and small intestine (correlating with fire), the middle finger reads the spleen and stomach (earth), and the ring finger reads the left kidney and reproductive organs (water). The physician's left hand then reads the right arm of the male patient. The index finger reads the lung and large intestine (metal), the middle finger reads the liver and gall bladder (wood), and the ring finger reads the right kidney and urinary bladder (water). If the patient is female the right arm is read first.

The three constitutional pulses are male, female, and neutral. The male pulse is thick and bulky, the female is thin and fast, and the neutral is smooth and supple. It is important for the physician to identify the constitutional pulse; otherwise it will be mistaken for the male as *rlung,* the female as *mkhris-pa,* and neutral as *bad-kan.*

The Tibetan astrological calendar has 360 days divided into spring, summer, autumn, and winter. Each has three months of thirty days. The first seventy-two days of spring (the first three months of the year) have a strong influence on the liver and gall bladder pulse, with wood predominating the season. This is followed by eighteen days with the earth element having special influence on the stomach and spleen pulse. The first seventy-two days of summer have a strong influence on the heart and small intestine pulses, with the fire element predominating the season. The first seventy-two days of autumn have a strong influence on the lungs and large intestine pulses, with metal predominant. Finally, the first seventy-two days of winter have a strong influence on the kidneys, urinary bladder, and reproductive organs pulses, with water predominant. For each of these last three seasons the earth element also predominates for the last eighteen days of each season. It is important for the physician to know the exact season when checking the pulse. Otherwise, in the summer, for example, the physician may confuse the stronger pulse of the heart and small intestine with disease. Because of the importance of seasons, medical texts describe how the physician can identify the seasons through observation of external changes of stars, birds, trees, and so on.

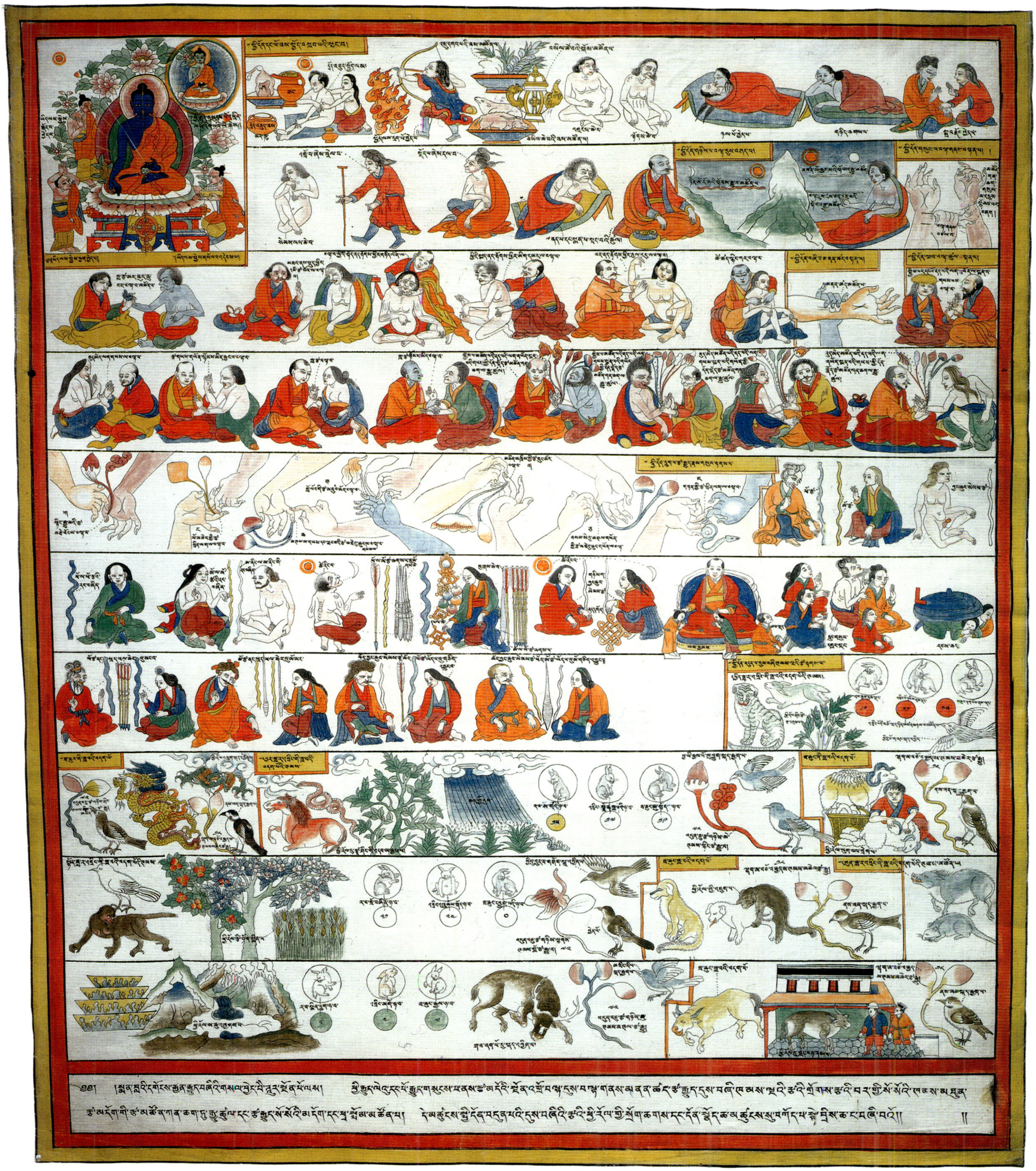

16. *Feeling the Pulse: Diagnosis and Divination*

This painting is a continuation from the previous one.

The wonder pulses (also called astonishing pulses) provide information about the patient's future and that of the patient's relatives. The pulses are divided into family prediction, guest prediction, enemy prediction, wealth prediction, demon prediction, substitutional pulse (read to obtain information about someone other than the person whose pulse is being read), and pregnancy predictions.

When the physician reads the pulse, its frequency will determine whether the patient is healthy or not. The frequency of the pulse is measured by the inhalation and exhalation of the physician. For healthy people, as the physician inhales the pulse should beat twice, in between inhalation and exhalation the pulse should beat once, and as the physician exhales, two more beats—five in total. This should be measured for a long time for accuracy. If the pulse is more than five the person has a hot disease, and if it is less than five the person has a cold disease.

Of the general pulses, there are hot pulses and cold pulses. A hot pulse is strong, overflowing, rolling, fast, twisted, and firm. A cold pulse is weak, sunken, declining, slow, loose, and empty. Six fingers of the physician can read the five full organs, the six hollow organs, and the upper and lower parts of the body.

With regard to the three *nyes-pas,* if it is a *rlung* disorder the pulse is floating, empty, and halting; if it is a *mkhris-pa* disorder the pulse is thin and twisted; and if it is a *bad-kan* disorder the pulse is slow and sunken.

If the patient has a blood disorder the pulse is bumpy and rolling. If it is a serum disorder the pulse is shaky and moves with difficulty. A leprosy pulse is trembling and thrilling. If the disorder is due to compounded poisons it is rough, short, and difficult to feel; if it is due to meat poisoning the pulse is thin, fast, sunken, or missing.

The death pulse is halting, irregular, changeable, or missing. If the heart pulse is missing the patient will live for one day; if the lung pulse is missing he will live for two days; if the liver pulse is missing he will live for three days; if the spleen pulse is missing he will live for five days; and if the kidney pulse is missing he will live for eight days.

Signs indicative of demonic possession are a sudden and erratic, concurrent, halting, and pulling pulse.

The pulse is read at the ulna artery to predict the lifespan of a healthy person. The ulna pulse should beat regularly and not be too strong or too weak. If the pulse beats continuously one hundred times it means the person will live for a hundred years; if it beats continuously fifty times the person will live for fifty years.

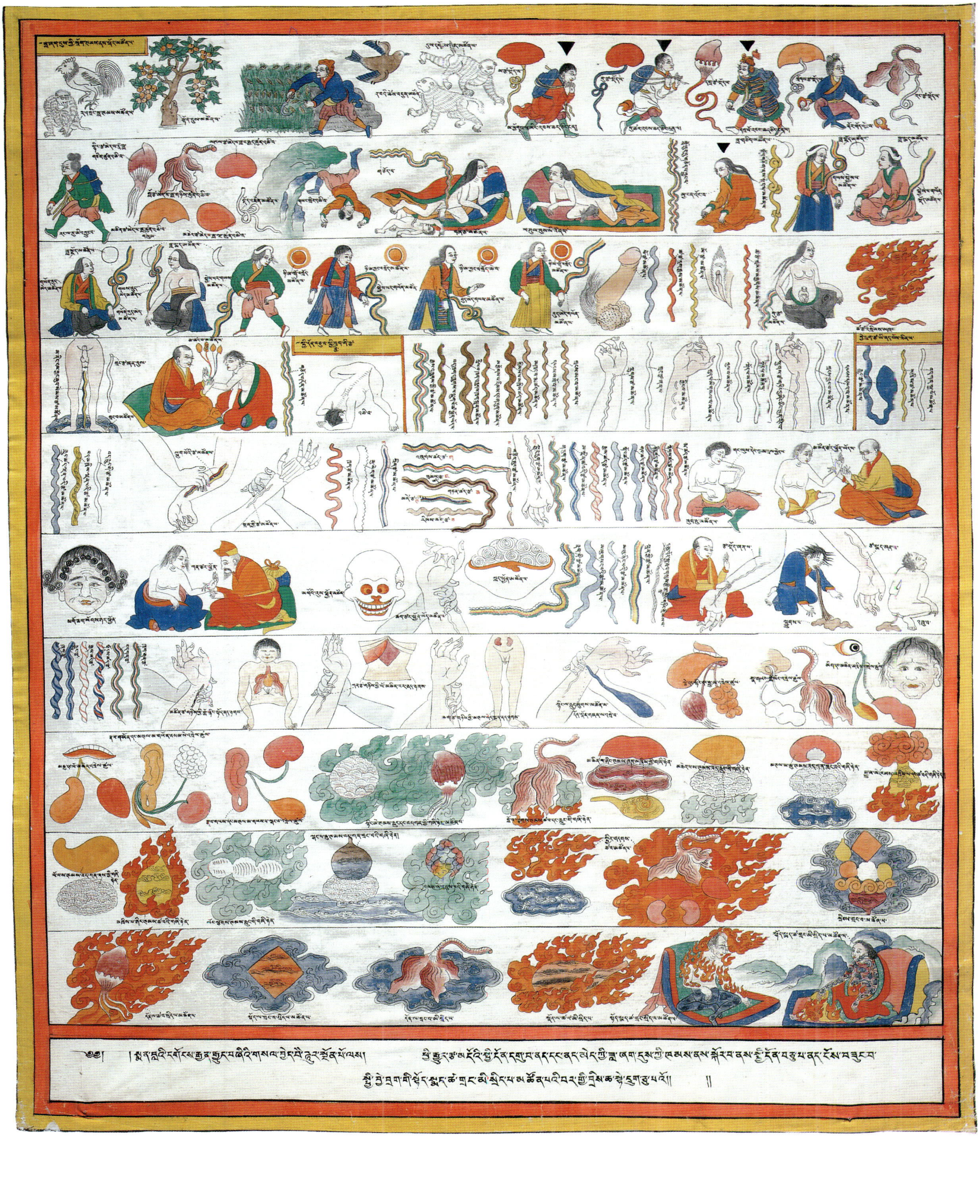
༄༅། །སྨན་བླའི་དགོངས་རྒྱན་རྒྱུད་པ་བཞིའི་གསལ་བྱེད་བཻ་ཌཱུར་སྔོན་པོ་ལས། ཕྱི་རྒྱུད་རྩ་མདོའི་སྤྱི་དོན་དགུ་པ་ནད་དང་ནད་མེད་ཀྱི་རྣ་ཞག་དུས་ཀྱི་ཁམས་ནས་སྐོར་བ་ནས་སྤྱི་དོན་བཅུ་པ་ནད་ངོས་བཟུང་བ
སྤྱི་ཏེ་བྲག་གི་ལྟོད་སྨད་ཆ་གྲང་མི་སྤྱོད་པ་མ་ཚོན་པའི་བར་གྱི་བྲིས་ཆ་སོ་དྲུག་རྩ་པའོ།། ||

17. Uroscopy: Diagnosis and Divination

For the Tibetan physician urine is like a mirror in which can be seen the internal imbalance of the patient, and his body temperature. This painting illustrates various conditions of the urine and exactly what disorders they indicate.

The night before uroscopy the patient should avoid drinking strong tea, buttermilk, and alcohol, as they may affect the color of the urine. The patient should also avoid sexual intercourse, mental stress, and physical exertion. The best analysis is taken from the first early-morning urine. The proper time for inspection is in the early-morning daylight to check color, vapor, and sediment. The best container to use for analysis is a white porcelain bowl that is not too shallow and not too deep, to accurately check the color of the urine.

It is important to understand how urine is formed, according to Tibetan medicine, so that the reasons for diagnoses are clear. Whatever we eat or drink goes into the stomach, where it is absorbed and digested. The waste products go through the small intestine to the large intestine, where they are separated into solid and liquid waste products. Liquid goes straight through the kidneys to the urethra and then to the urinary bladder. The essence of food goes to the liver and produces blood; the impurities in the blood go to the gall bladder and produce bile. The essence of bile produces serum, and the impurities in the bile become the sediments in the urine. Because of these factors the intake of food can affect the color of urine. It is also possible to read body temperature by observing the thickness of the sediments.

A healthy person's urine is light yellow like melted butter. The vapors are not too strong or weak. The urine has medium-sized bubbles, the sediment is of average density, and the urine is clear.

When the urine is freshly collected and still hot, the physician checks the color, vapor, odor, and bubbles. As the urine cools, the physician checks the sediments and scum. When the urine is cold, it is stirred and the physician checks to see how long it takes for the bubbles to disperse and the way the bubbles are dispersed. After that the physician checks to see if the color of the urine has changed.

If the patient is suffering from a *rlung* disease, the urine is blueish, with little vapor and odor, and big bubbles. If it is a *mkhris-pa* disease the urine is yellow, with a strong odor and vapor, and the bubbles will disperse very quickly. If it is a *bad-kan* disease the urine is white, with little odor and vapor, and steady bubbles.

If the urine is blackish and rainbow-colored the disease has been caused by poison. If the sediment is like sand the patient has a kidney disorder. If it is like a cloud the patient has a lung disorder. If there is scum on the urine that separates into small pieces, the patient has a tumor problem.

When the urine is like blood, its odor like rotten leather, sour milk, or expired ink, it is a sign of impending death. Likewise if the urine is blue, there is no odor or vapor, and the physician observes no changes in the bubbles after checking the urine.

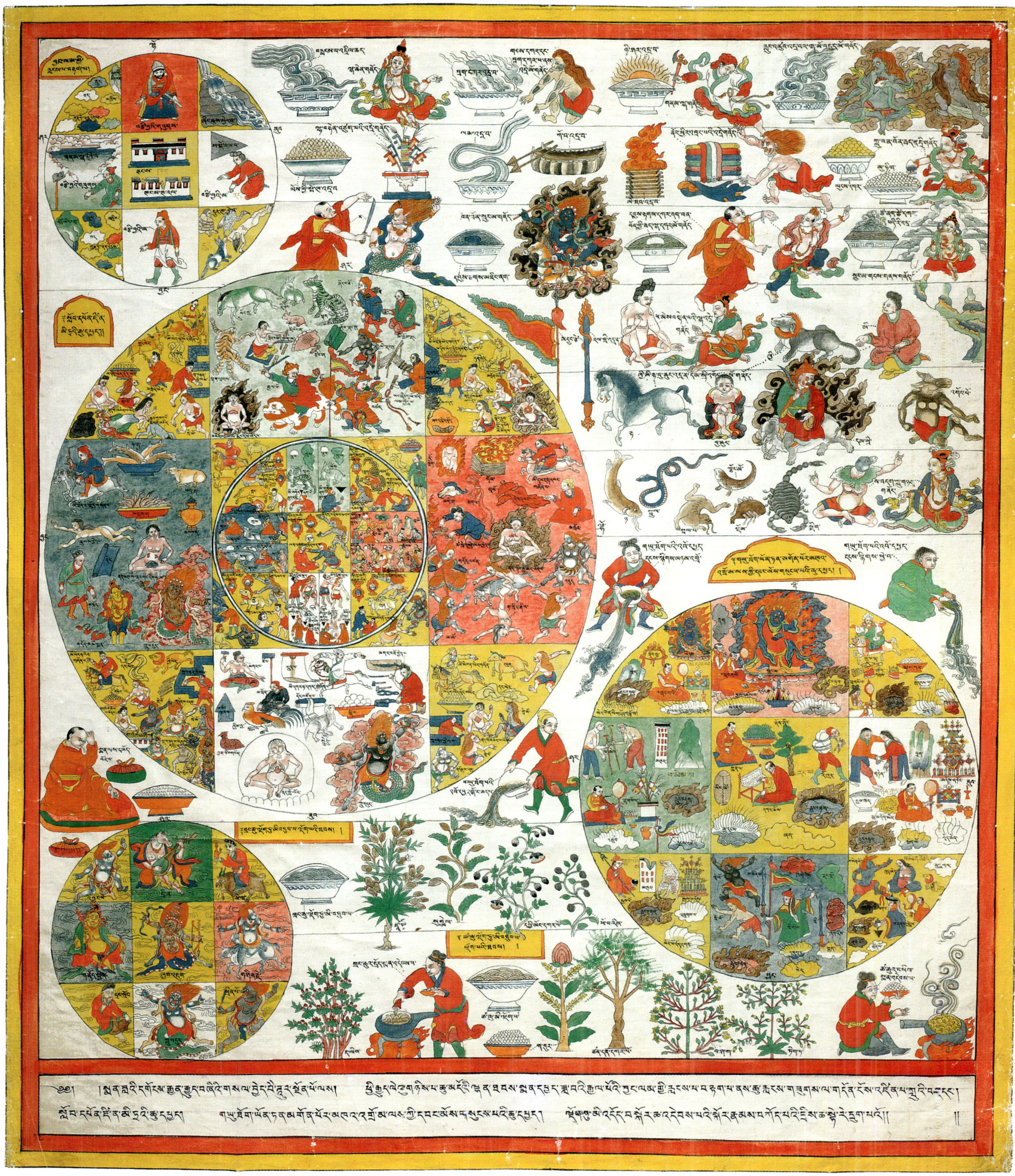

18. *Uroscopy: Diagnosis and Divination*

This painting is a continuation from the preceding painting (plate 17) and it shows the diagnosis of demonic possession through analyzing urine. Within the Tibetan view, imbalance of the three *nyes-pas* of *rlung, mkhris-pa,* and *bad-kan* is often caused by spirits and demons. Since many of the consequent illnesses may be severe, it is important to determine the class of offending demon, so that rituals of appeasement may commence.

When the physician collects the patient's urine in a container, the container should be visualized as a tortoise sleeping on its back, with its head pointing north and its tail pointing south. The urine in the container is then divided into nine sectors with two vertical and two horizontal thin wooden sticks. The right three sectors of this division represent gods, humans, and demons; the left three sectors represent cemetery, house, and agriculture; and the middle three sectors are maternal ancestors, patient, and son/nephew.

The physician then looks for any images, bubbles, sediments, or scum in any of the sectors.

If anything is seen in the gods sector it means the god is disturbed, and prayers will have to be performed. If anything is seen in the human sector it is associated with male and female demons who have caused the patient's illness, and rituals have to be performed to banish them. If anything is seen in the demon sector, thread-cross[1] and exorcisms will have to be performed. If anything is seen in cemetery, house, or agriculture sectors, local deities and *nagas* will have to be propitiated by offering milk and incense, and by performing treasure vase offerings. If anything is seen in the maternal ancestor sector it means that demons have appeared through attachment to property, and *torma* (a ritual cake made of barley) will have to be offered. If anything is seen in the patient sector it means that the patient has mixed their clothes with those of their friends or lovers, and the demonic influence comes through the clothes; the clothes will therefore have to be destroyed. If anything is seen in the son/nephew square the spirit comes from the patient's uncle, mother, or aunt. An effigy will have to be made and pointed in the direction of the uncle, mother, or aunt.

There are other systems of uroscopy such as that of Master Jinamitra, which divides the urine sample into twelve sectors that are linked to the twelve signs of the Tibetan zodiac: tiger, hare, dragon, snake, horse, sheep, monkey, bird, dog, pig, mouse, and bull. In the *King of the Moon* treatise the urine sample is divided into nine sectors and then subdivided into the four cardinal directions, which are then linked to the four elements and the four seasons. This treatise was written by Yuthog Yontan Gonpo the Younger (the founder of Tibetan medicine), who received it from the *dakini* Karmamahendrani. The nine sectors are analyzed according to positive signs, negative signs, saliva divination, *rlung* signs, *mkhris-pa* signs, and *bad-kan* signs.

Uroscopy, especially with regard to demonic possession, is one of the most complicated aspects of Tibetan medicine.

1. A ritual procedure used in Bon, the ancient pre-Buddhist religion of Tibet, in which threads are strung across the patient's body in order to detect spirits who cause illness.

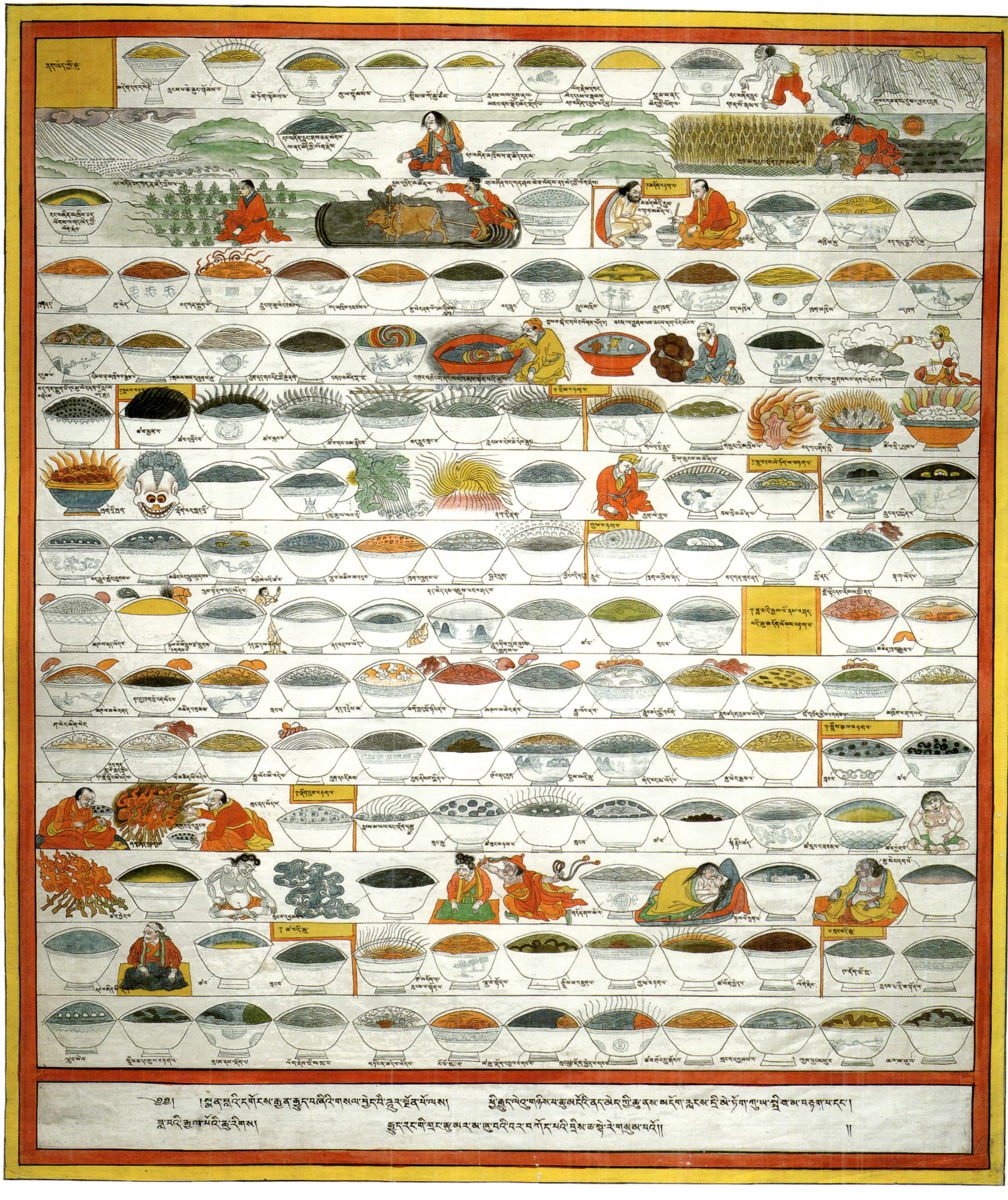

19. *The Tree of Treatment*

This painting shows that once an imbalance of *rlung, mkhris-pa,* and *bad-kan* is accurately diagnosed, treatment can begin.

The root of treatment has four trunks (from left to right): advice on diet, advice on conduct, prescribing medicine, and performing external therapies.

Advice on diet has branches for *rlung, mkhris-pa,* and *bad-kan.* The nature of *rlung* is light and rough; an imbalance is counteracted by recommending oily and nutritious foods such as molasses, butter, garlic, onion, meat, milk, mustard oil for cooking, soup, and alcohol in moderation. The nature of *mkhris-pa* is hot and sharp; an imbalance is counteracted by recommending cool and light foods such as cow and goat milk, yogurt and buttermilk, goat meat, vegetables, nongreasy foods, and water. The nature of *bad-kan* is cold; an imbalance is counteracted by recommending a warming diet of lamb, yak meat, honey, barley, hot water, *dri's* (female yak) milk curd, and buttermilk.

Advice on conduct: A *rlung* patient should live in a dim and warm apartment, and enjoy the company of friends and lovers. A *mkhris-pa* patient should live in a cool place, preferably by the sea, and get plenty of rest. A *bad-kan* patient should exercise regularly and live in a warm, sunny, and cozy apartment.

Prescribing medicine: For a *rlung* patient medicine with sweet, sour, salty, heavy, and smooth taste and potency is prescribed. For a *mkhris-pa* patient medicine with sweet, bitter, astringent, cool, and blunt taste and potency is prescribed. For a *bad-kan* patient medicine with hot, sour, astringent, sharp, coarse, and light taste and potency is prescribed.

Performing external therapies: For a *rlung* patient therapies include mild enemas, massages, or hot oil compresses on the various points of *rlung*—the sternum, crown of the head, palms, and the soles of the feet. For a *mkhris-pa* patient the doctor might perform mild purgative therapies, cooling therapies such as placing the patient beneath a waterfall, or bloodletting at various points of the body. For a *bad-kan* patient the doctor might induce vomiting or perform moxibustion.

This is only a brief explanation of treatment methods; in fact there are ninety-eight different methods of treatment for imbalances in the three *nyes-pas.* If the physician applies full concentration and effort he will be able to pull the patient safely from the swamp of illness.

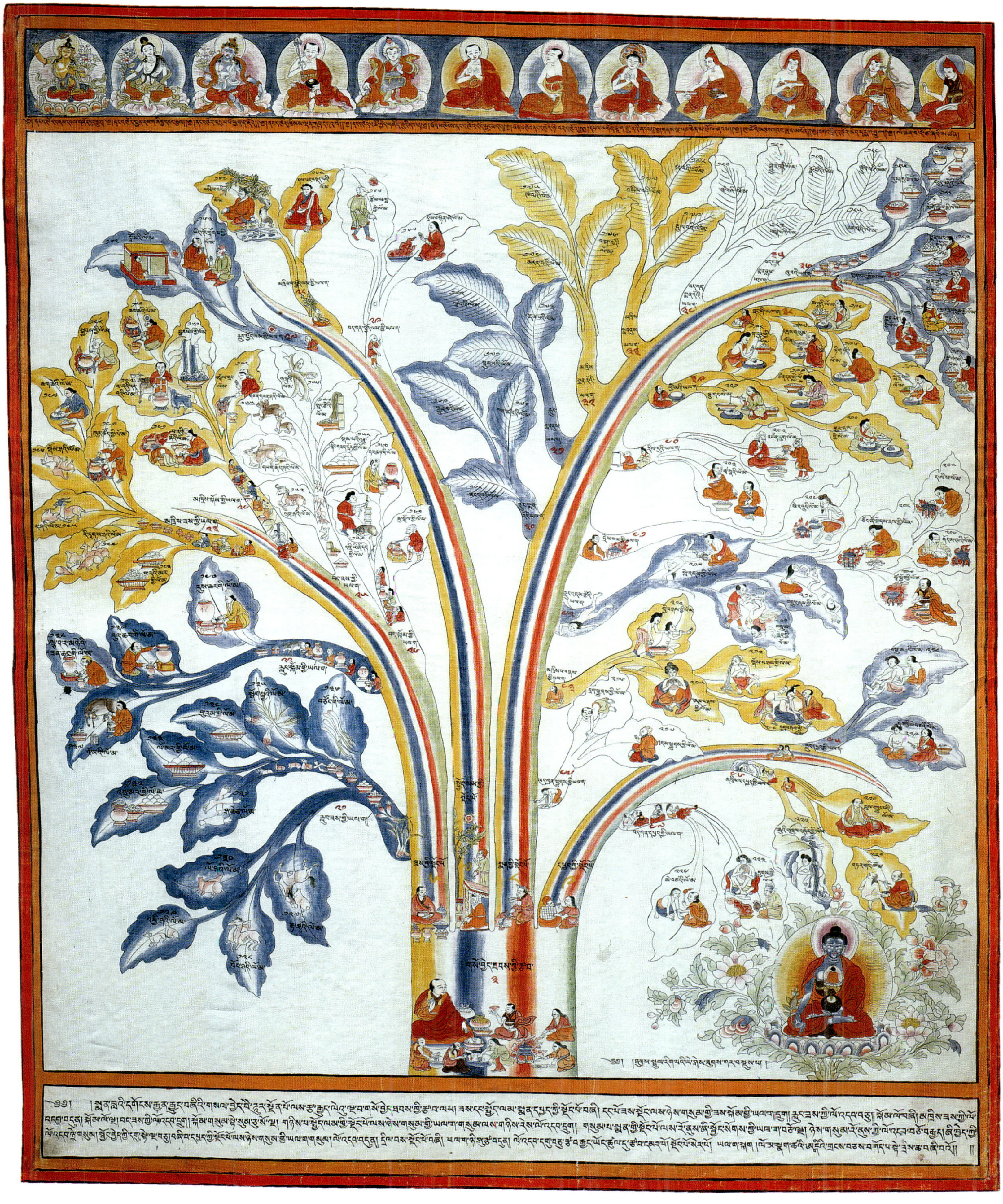

20. General Therapeutic Principles

This painting shows how to lead a healthy life by maintaining a balanced diet, following proper conduct, and using the right medicine.

All diseases can be placed into two categories—hot diseases and cold diseases. The diagnostic process consists of visual inspection, palpation, and questioning (illustrated on the right side of the second row).

The key items to check in an examination are the five sense organs, urine, sputum, vomit, feces, and blood.

Visual inspection includes checking skin color, body shape and size, and other things that the physician can see with the naked eye.

Palpation consists of reading the pulse, feeling the body temperature, and feeling the roughness or smoothness of the skin. The pulse is like a messenger between the physician and the patient. Through experience and knowledge the physician is able to read many different pulses.

Questioning is also a useful and informative diagnostic technique. It involves listening to the patient describe symptoms, location of illness, and causative factors. Correct diagnosis requires careful observation, experience, and listening.

Once a diagnosis has been made there are four levels of a disease's seriousness with regard to the possibilities of success in treatment: some are easily treatable, some difficult to treat, some with a remote chance of a cure, and some that are incurable or not to be cured for various reasons. For an illness that is easily cured, we simply need a good physician, good medicine, caring nursing, and an obedient patient. Illnesses that are difficult to cure are chronic diseases that need many different methods of treatment over a long period of time. If the patient does not have a good physician and good nursing, the disease will be difficult to cure. For diseases that have a remote chance of a cure, we can see that some patients are diagnosed as incurable, though the patients may remain alive for a long time. This is because, as Buddhists, Tibetans believe that an individual's own lifespan is based on karma. For some people this can be as short as one week and for others as long as a hundred years. Diseases are incurable when the patient is unable to take food and drink, and when there are only skin and bones, no pulse, and no response to any form of treatment. For the physician to withhold treatment the patient would have to be particularly evil—someone who would only commit many negative and harmful actions to society if they remained alive.

There are ten ways of taking medicine. If it is a *bad-kan* disorder, the medicine should be taken on an empty stomach and in the early morning. If the disease is connected with downward-cleansing *rlung*, the medicine should be taken immediately before lunch. If it is a *rlung* disorder, medicine must be taken during lunch. If it is a pervasive *rlung* disorder, medicine should be taken immediately after lunch or dinner. If it is a life-sustaining *rlung* disorder, medicine should be taken in small doses and at the same time as eating food, a little after every alternate mouthful. If it is an upward-moving *rlung* disorder, medicine should be taken as soon as food has been digested. If the patient has asthma, medicine should be taken in small doses and as frequently as possible. If the patient has a weak appetite, medicine is taken with food. If the patient suffers from hiccups, medicine should be taken both before and after meals. If the patient has diseases connected to the head, medicine should be taken before dinner and after food has been digested.

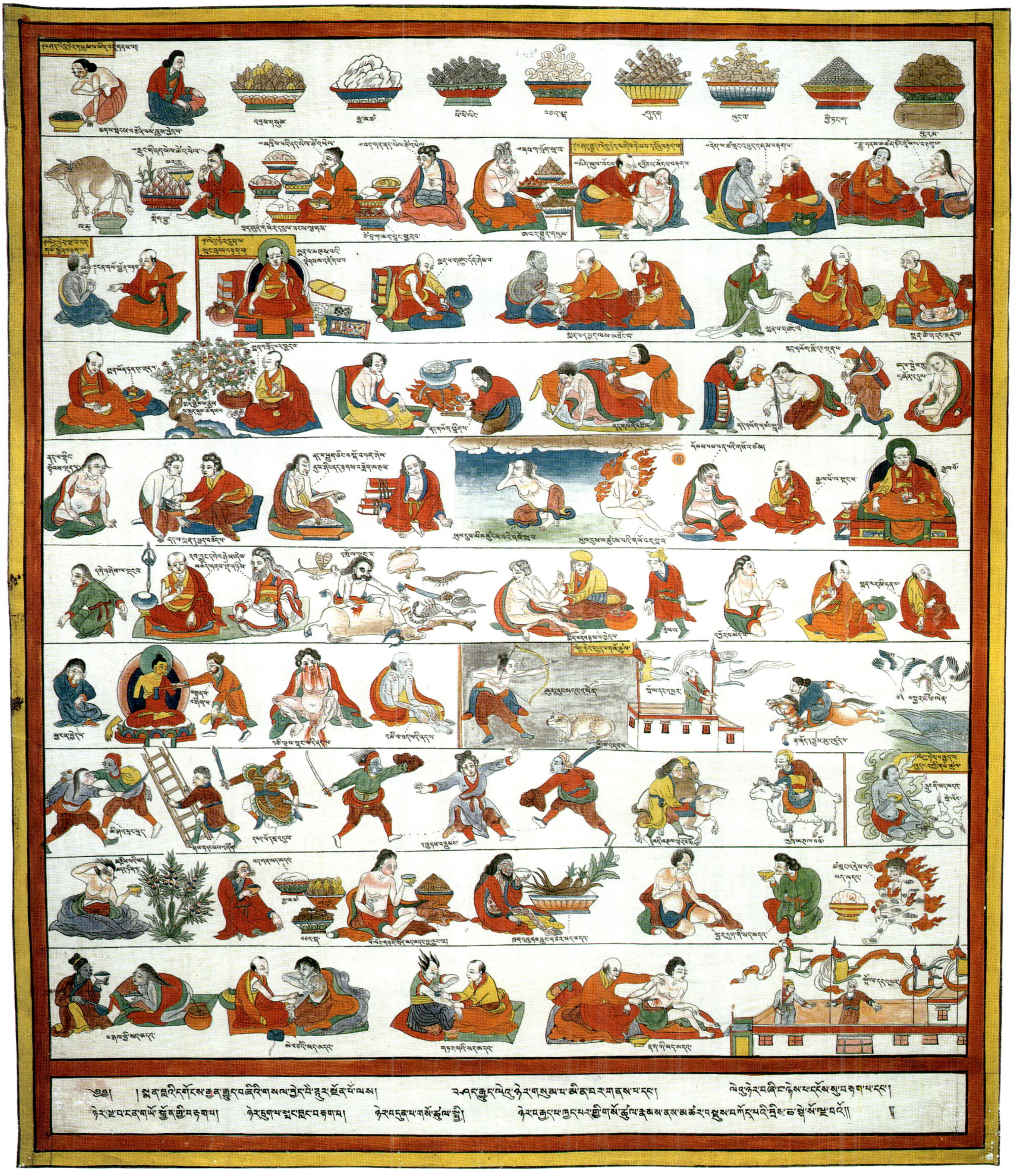

21. *Conduct*

In Tibetan medicine conduct is divided into daily, occasional, and seasonal conduct. The following rules should be observed in one's daily conduct:

1. *do not kill other beings;*
2. *avoid sexual misconduct such as adultery or having sex with a partner in front of sacred images;*
3. *do not take what is not yours;*
4. *do not lie;*
5. *do not gossip;*
6. *do not verbally abuse or slander anyone;*
7. *do not engage in divisive talk;*
8. *do not be covetous;*
9. *do not be intentionally harmful; and*
10. *do not hold erroneous or perverted views.*

With regard to money, when you save, save well, and when you spend be generous. If you win something you should know your limit. If you did something wrong admit it. Be friendly with people and remember the kindness shown to you by friends and relatives; respect your parents and elders. Always try to assist those afflicted by sorrow or mental suffering, disabled people, the destitute, and beggars; never look down on those less fortunate. Regard all beings as the same as oneself. With regard to actions, do things at the right time. With regard to sex, it is good to have as much as you desire in the winter, every two days in the spring and autumn, and once every fortnight in the summer; too much sex can weaken the whole system, especially the eyes.

Tibetan Buddhists also believe in spiritual power, and such things as wearing blessing threads for protection, and gold and diamonds to prolong life and overcome obstacles.

Concerning occasional conduct, one should not suppress certain natural bodily functions—hunger, yawning, sneezing, vomiting, breathing, sleeping, expectorant phlegm, salivation, flatulence, urination, and ejaculation.

Concerning seasonal conduct, the internal five elements and the external five elements are connected, so we have to behave in accordance with the change of seasons.

In winter one should have massages with sesame oil, eat nutritious foods such as meat broth and soup, wear warm clothes such as wool, and sit near fires, not getting too cold.

In spring one should eat honey and drink a lot of hot water, one should have food and drink such as ginger decoction, barley, and beef, and one should exercise frequently and have massages with pea flour.

In a dry summer one should eat light, sweet, and cooling foods such as rice, beef, and vegetables. One should avoid direct sunshine and take cool baths. One can also drink alcohol mixed with spring water, wear light clothes, and enjoy cool breezes and sit in the shade.

In a wet summer one should drink buttermilk and eat foods that generate digestive heat, such as garlic, ginger, cinnamon, and nutmeg.

In autumn one should eat sweet, bitter, and astringent foods, and wear clothes scented with sandalwood and camphor.

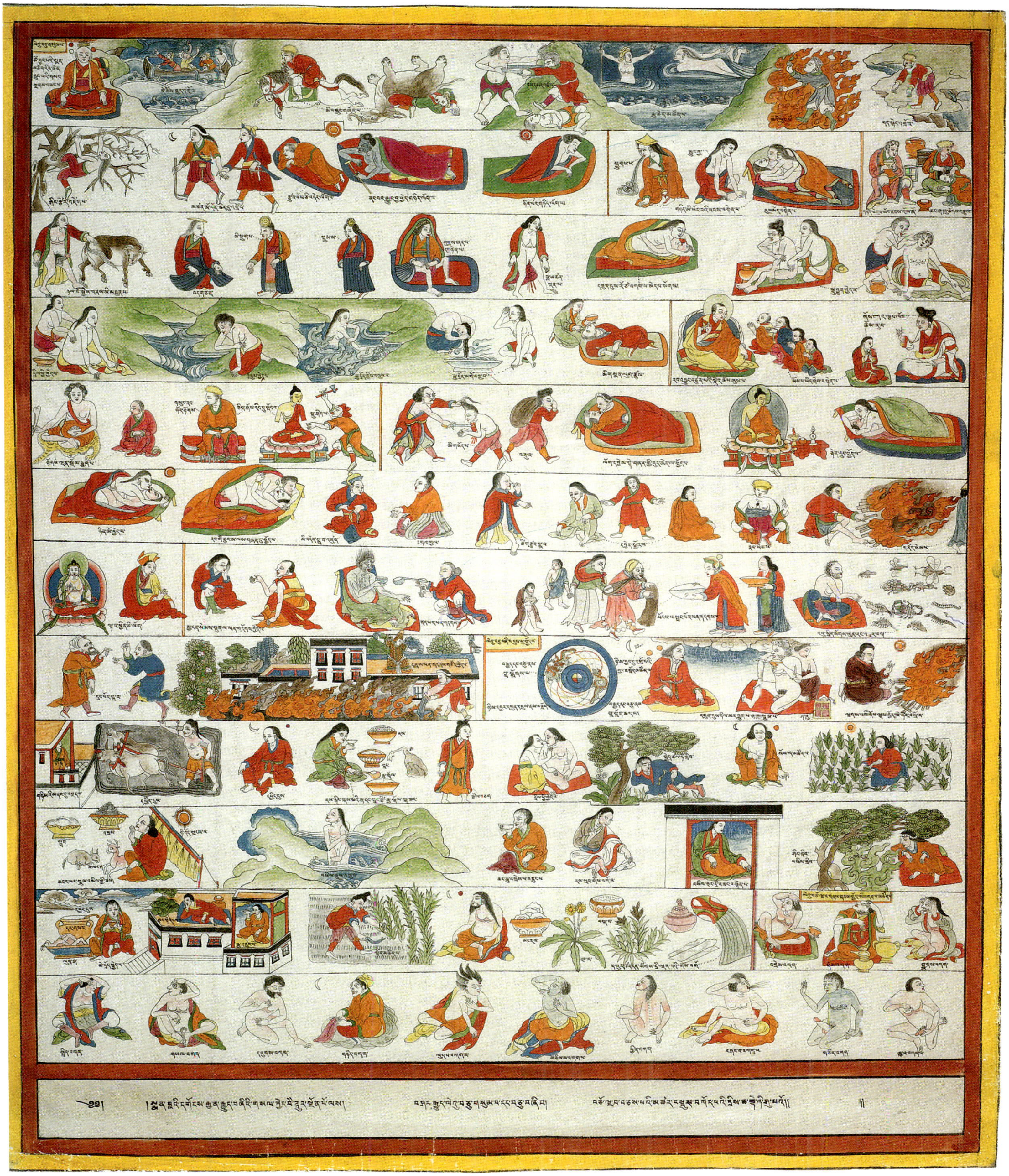

22. *Diet*

This painting shows the importance in Tibetan medicine of a proper balanced diet. It is divided into food and drink.

Food is divided into five categories: grains, meat, oil, vegetables, and cooked foods.

Grain is divided into cereals and pulses. Cereals include rice, millet, oats, wheat, and barley. The most nutritious is barley, and rice is the easiest to digest; it stops diarrhea and vomiting, and it increases virility. Pulses include peas, black and white beans, lentils, mung beans, linseed, sesame seeds, and buckwheat. Lentils are the easiest to digest, and the application of powdered lentils can help ringworm and gout. All cereals should be fully ripened and well cooked; pulses should be soaked overnight and then cooked.

Meat includes chicken, rabbit, buffalo, yak, *dzo,*[1] horse, beef, goat, lamb, duck, pork, fish, and crab. Fish improves the digestive heat, appetite, eyesight, tumors, wounds, and memory. Buffalo meat increases weight and aids sleep. Rabbit increases the digestive heat and stops diarrhea. Crab is good for the kidneys and water retention. All meats should be thoroughly cooked.

Oil includes butter, mustard oil, sesame oil, bone marrow oil, and animal fat. Butter is good for virility, the complexion, the digestive system, to heal wounds, and to improve the memory.

In Tibet there were not many vegetables so the examples given are few: garlic, onion, chiles, ginger, radish, dandelion, turnip, marsh mallow, rhubarb, and nettles. Garlic has a hot potency and is good for eliminating worms; it increases body heat, and is good for insomnia. Ginger helps warm the body, helps blood circulation, and is good for the appetite. Chiles have a warm potency and are good for the digestive system and the appetite. Radish improves the digestive heat.

Cooked food includes porridges made from rice, meat, milk and rice, barley, and wheat. The most nutritious porridge is *tsampa,* made from ground roasted barley; it is the staple food of Tibetans.

Drink is divided into milk, water, and alcohol.

Milk includes cows' milk, goats' milk, and sheep's milk. Also included in this group are buttermilk and yogurt. Cows' milk is good for the lungs, diabetes, and chronic colds; goats' milk is good for asthma; sheep's milk is heavy, and bad for the heart. Yogurt is good for the appetite but it can cause constipation; buttermilk increases digestive heat and reduces tumors and piles.

There are seven types of water, illustrated in the center of the painting: rain, glacial, river, spring, well, sea, and forest. Of these rainwater is the best, like nectar. In Tibetan medical texts, boiled hot water has many benefits—it helps digestion of fatty foods, reduces gas formation, and helps asthma, colds, and flu.

Alcohol—called *chang* in Tibet—is made from fermented wheat, barley, millet, and rice. The taste is sour and bitter; it can cause diarrhea, increase body heat and sleepiness, and cause people to become more confident and relaxed. Drinking too much can cause problems. In Tibetan medicine drunkenness has three stages, illustrated in the eighth row. First, people become more talkative and their behavior changes; there is a lack of conscience and general shamelessness. A Tibetan proverb says that alcohol is the key to unlock the shy person's mouth. The second stage is the most dangerous stage, when people start fighting, crying, and harming others. This stage is compared to a mad elephant. The third stage is when people are so drunk they are unable to remember anything. Therefore it is very important to drink in the right quantity.

To consume food in moderate quantities, depending on the consistency of the food, is essential. If it is a heavy food such as lamb, fill only half of your stomach; if it is a light food such as rice,

1. A crossbreed: part bull and part female yak.

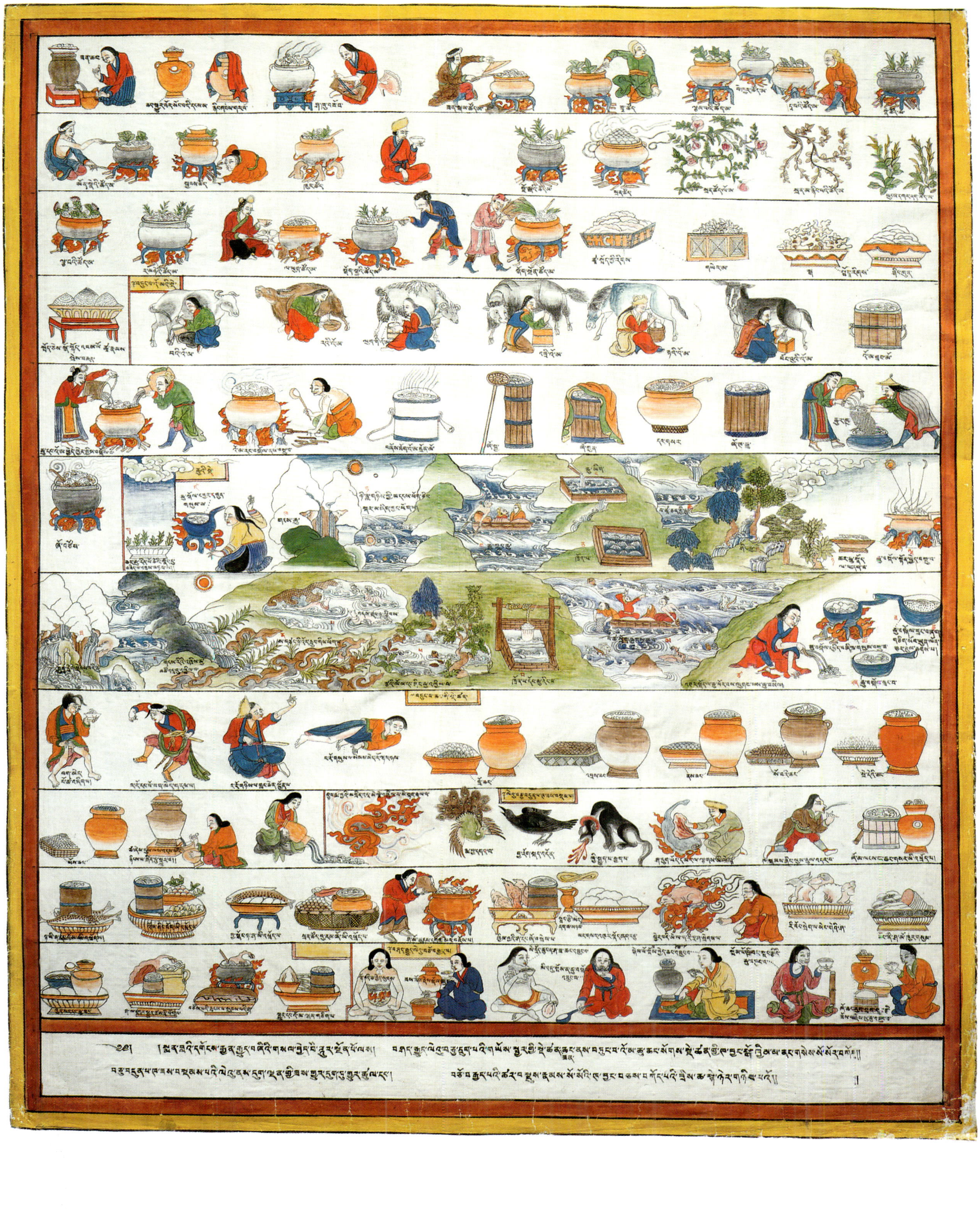

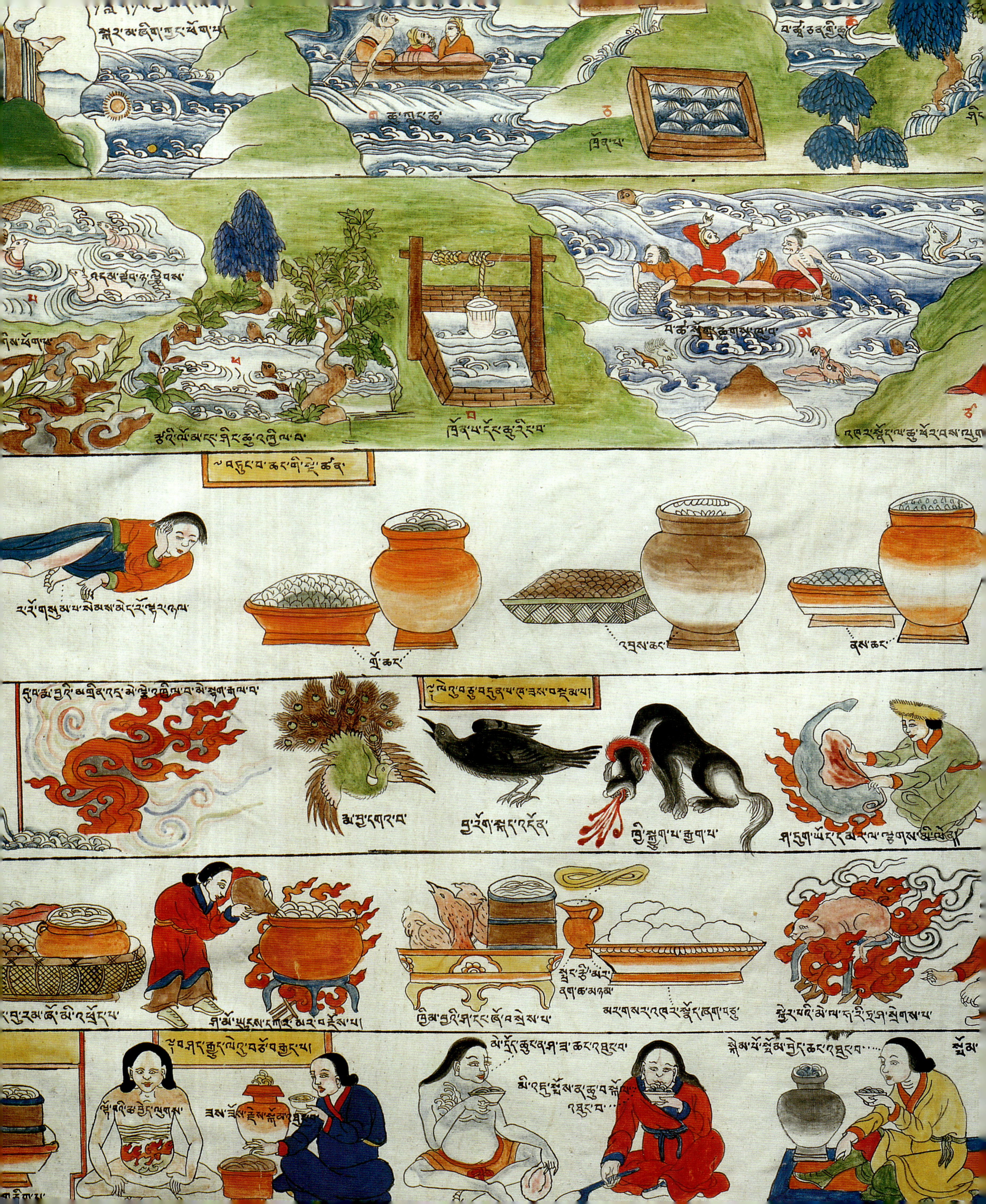

you can fill yourself up more. Your stomach must feel comfortable for the food to be easily digested. It is important to visualize your stomach in four parts: two parts for solid food, a third part for liquids, and a fourth part for space. It is also important to drink liquid after eating, and if you have indigestion drink hot boiling water. If you eat sensibly you will have a healthy life.

In Tibetan medicine the digestive system is the most important part of our body because whatever we eat or drink has to be absorbed. The decomposing *bad-kan* helps to break down solid foods into a semiliquid state in the stomach. Then the digestive *mkhris-pa,* located between the stomach and intestine, further helps to digest the food. Finally, the fire-accompanying *rlung* separates the liquid in our stomach and intestine into nutrients and waste products. The essence of nutrients goes to the liver to form blood, which forms muscle tissue, which forms bones, which form bone marrow, which forms generative fluid. The waste products go to the colon and separate into feces and urine. The feces goes to the rectum and the urine goes through the urethra to the kidneys and the urinary bladder.

Overeating causes an increase of mucus in the stomach. Excess mucus can block the channels, disturbing the digestive process. This is the cause of all digestive illnesses. It is therefore very important to eat sensibly.

Dietary restrictions cover food poisons and incompatible foods (illustrated in the last two rows). Poisonous food is identified by unnatural taste and color. If the poisonous food is burned, the smoke that appears will be as blue as a peacock's neck, and the flame does not go upward but sways to one side. If the food has been deliberately poisoned, the poisoner will look nervous, restless, and will be sweating. Poisonous food should be buried underground. Incompatible foods can also harm us. Combinations such as chicken and yogurt, fish and milk, or milk and fruit are incompatible, and when eaten together might lead to digestive problems. When trying new foods that you have not tasted before, it is best to eat only a little in the beginning, in order to allow your body to become used to it.

23. *Poisons*

This painting shows the three different types of poisons: compounded poisons, food poisons, and naturally grown poisons. The creature in the center is called Kalakuta or Halahala, poison incarnate.

According to prophecies in the Tibetan medical texts the age in which we now live is a time when the world's natural resources are being depleted; there is a great disruption in the environment and the five natural elements. These factors create the causes for eighteen new types of malignant diseases that threaten the lives of humans.

Compounded poison can be a combination of precious stones and metals such as gold, silver, copper, bronze, iron, lead, and mercury; and minerals such as iron hydroxide, iron ore, zinc, calcite, and sulphur. Such combinations can produce poison that is then transmitted through the rays of the sun, smoke, polluted air, physical touch, and contaminated food.

Food poisons are caused by the combination of incompatible foods (see plate 22). Also, eating something that one is not used to can upset the digestive system and disrupt the seven bodily constituents and three excretory functions.

Naturally grown poisons include plant poisons and animal poisons. The painting identifies poisonous plants such as black and yellow aconite *(Aconitum ferux Wall)*, datura, caltrops, spurge *(Euphorbia)*, and madar grass *(Caltropis gigantea)*. Snake venom, the bite of a rabid dog, and scorpion and bee stings are examples of animal poisons.

If someone accidentally took aconite the symptoms would be numbness in the tongue and limbs, a burning sensation, cracked lips and tongue, black complexion, cold breath, fainting, loss of consciousness, stiffness in the limbs, and a bloated stomach with excruciating pain. The physician would immediately give a herbal combination of natron, tumeric, and myrobalan *(Terminalia chebula)* to prevent the spread of the poison.

If someone is bitten by a rabid dog (the dog will look deaf and blind, saliva will be running from its mouth, its head will be bent, its tail inverted, and it will wander aimlessly) the person's wound turns black and brown and becomes swollen. If it is not treated immediately the patient gets headaches, chills, and becomes delirious, faints, pants, and is unable to look in a mirror or in water. When the disease is advanced the human behaves like a dog. For rabies, the physician purges toxins from the system by prescribing medicine such as a great multi-compounded Precious Pill, or a great cold-compounded black Precious Pill. These pills contain more than seventy different types of minerals and herbs as an antidote to the poison. Also, spiritual help from an advanced tantric practitioner can be used, or the poisons can be sucked out of the wound if treatment is sought immediately.

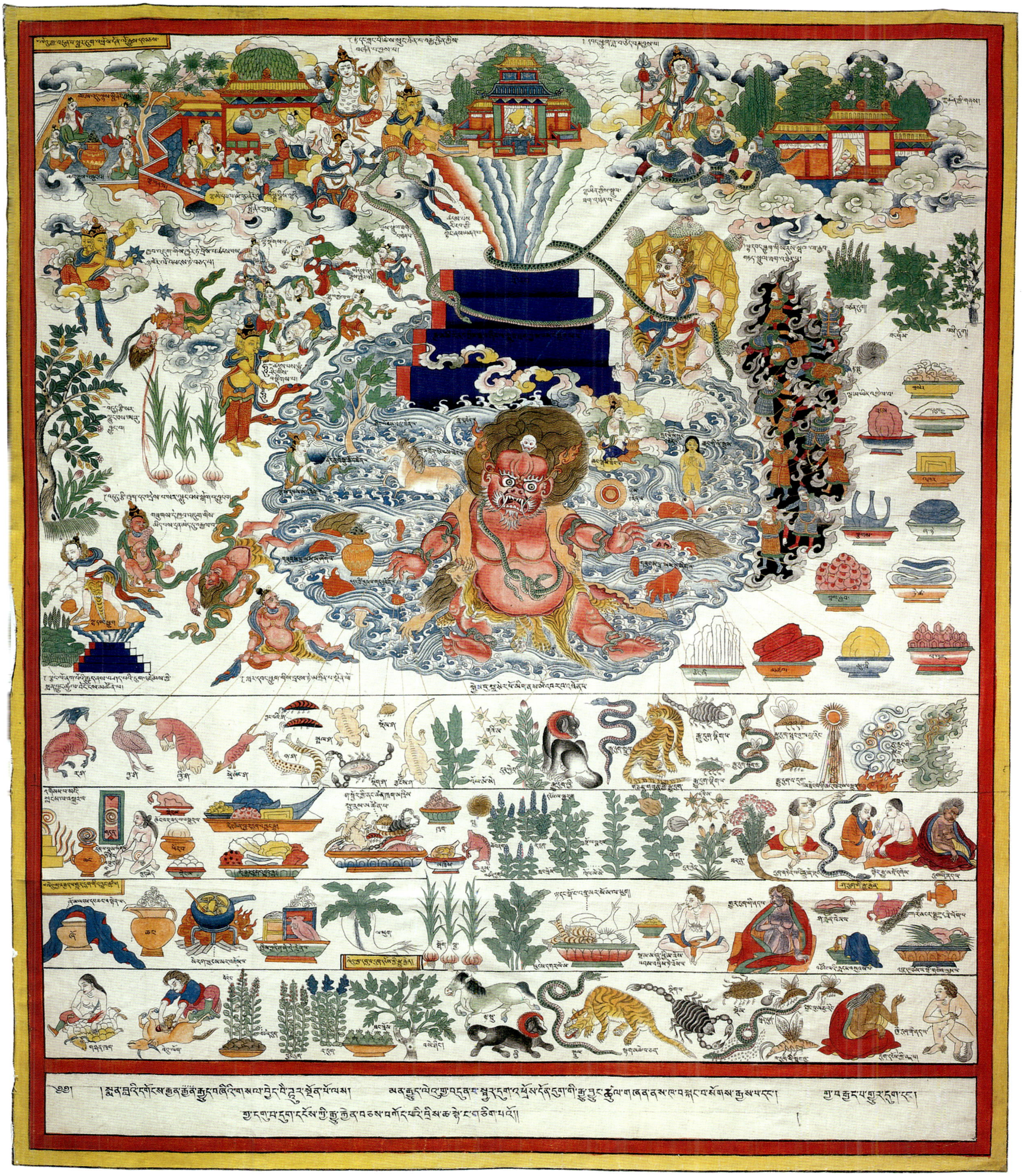

24. *Materia Medica of Mineral Origin*

This painting shows the eight classifications of ingredients used in the preparation of Tibetan medicine: 1. precious gemstones and metals; 2. soils; 3. minerals; 4. wood; 5. nectars; 6. shrubs grown in hot plains climate; 7. herbs; and 8. animal products.

The compounding methods of Tibetan medicines are either a combination of tastes, potencies, or post-digestive tastes (resulting from the digestive process).

Medicines that are combinations of sweet, sour, salty, and hot tastes will help eliminate excess *rlung*. Medicines combining bitter, sweet, and astringent tastes will help eliminate excess *mkhris-pa*. Medicines combining hot, sour, and salty tastes will help eliminate excess *bad-kan*.

Most Tibetan medicinal preparations, however, are combinations of the eight potencies—heavy/light, hot/cold, oily/rough, and dull/sharp. These eight potencies can be divided into the seventeen qualities that can counteract the subtle natures of *rlung, mkhris-pa,* and *bad-kan*.

Earth has the following qualities: heavy, stable, blunt, smooth, oily, and dry. These qualities pacify *rlung* disorders, because the nature of *rlung* is light, movable, cool, rough, hard, and thin. Earth can aggravate *bad-kan* because they share the same qualities.

Water has the following qualities: fluidity, cooling, heavy, blunt, oily, and supple. These qualities pacify *mkhris-pa* disorders, because the nature of *mkhris-pa* is oily, pungent, hot, light, sharp, and moist. Water can aggravate *bad-kan* because they share the same qualities.

Fire has the following qualities: hot, sharp, dry, coarse, light, oily, and mobile. These qualities pacify *bad-kan* disorders, because the nature of *bad-kan* is cool, blunt, smooth, sticky, heavy, steady, and oily. Fire can aggravate *mkhris-pa* because they share the same qualities.

Air has the following qualities: light, mobile, cold, coarse, pale, and dry. These qualities pacify *bad-kan* disorders. Air can aggravate *rlung* because they share the same qualities.

The main gemstones and precious metals used in Tibetan medicine are pearl, coral, turquoise, lapis, sapphire, diamond, achates, emerald, ruby, gold, silver, iron, and copper. All the gemstones and minerals have to be detoxified, refined, and powdered before they can be used as medicine.

Of the gems, turquoise has an astringent taste and cool potency. It treats hepatitis and eye disease, and it is an antidote. Pearl has an astringent taste and cool potency. It treats brain damage due to inflammation or injury, nerve degeneration, stiffness and contraction of ligaments and tendons, paralysis, and it is an antidote. Lapis has an astringent taste and cool potency. It is an antidote, treating skin diseases, leprosy, and premature graying of hair. Achate, another precious stone, has an astringent taste and cool potency, treating epilepsy, headaches, and eye diseases. Emerald has an astringent taste and cool potency, treating epilepsy and neurological diseases; they are also an antipyretic.

Of the precious metals, gold has an astringent taste and cool potency. It promotes longevity and rejuvenation, and counteracts oxide poisons. Iron has an astringent taste and cool potency. It treats eye diseases and edema, and alleviates poisoning of the liver.

Minerals used include orpiment, charcoal, stalactite, limestone, zinc, marcasite, hematite, and tourmaline. Of the minerals, limestone has a sweet taste and hot potency, and stops diarrhea, eliminates fever, and strengthens bones and the digestive system. Realgar has a bitter taste and hot potency, and relieves glandular fever and septic wounds. Stalactite has an astringent taste and hot potency, and strengthens the tendons and ligaments weakened due to injury. Hematite has an astringent taste and cool potency, and heals cracks, bone fractures, and brain damage due to accidents. Charcoal dissolves stones and stops bleeding.

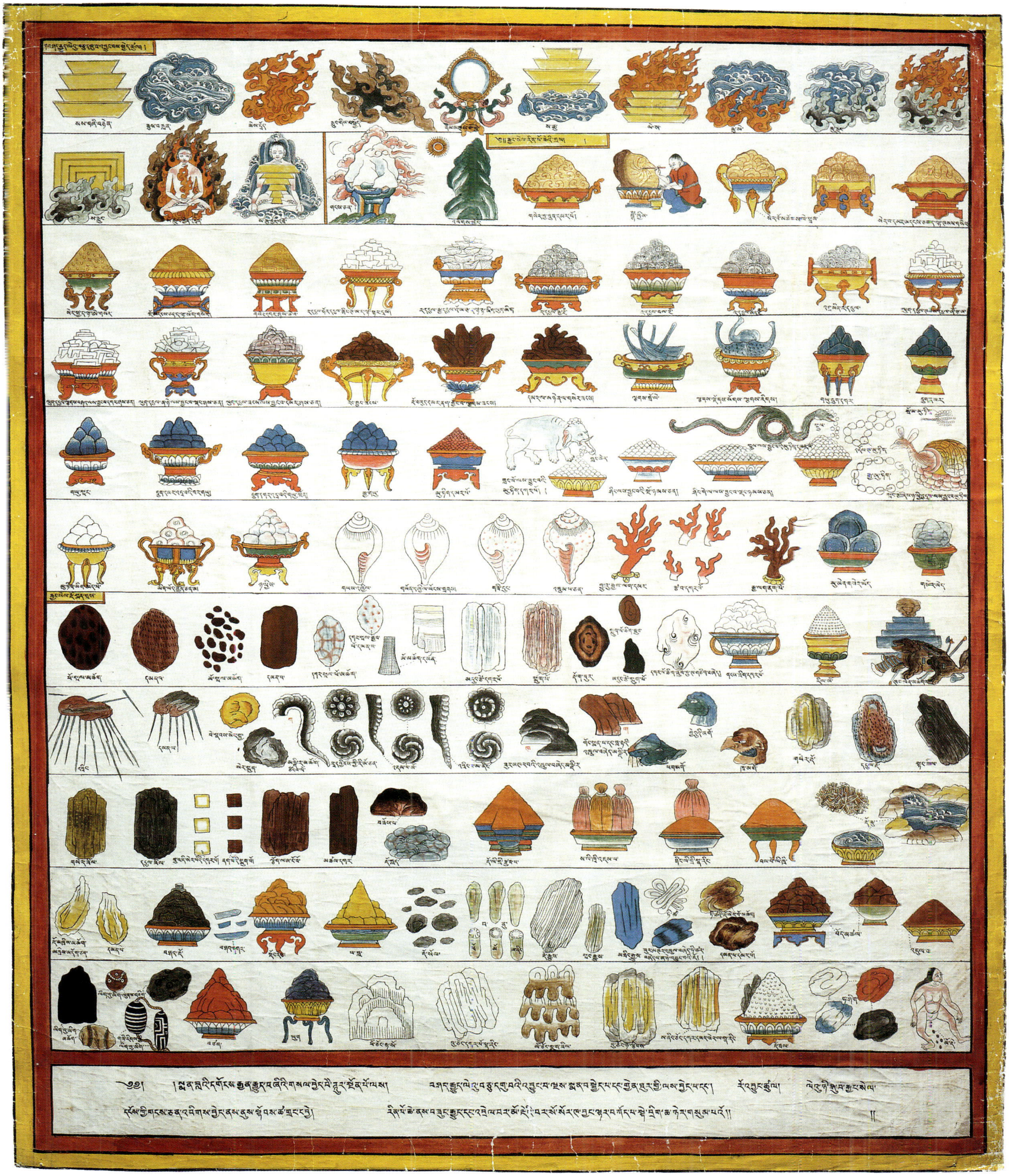

25. *Materia Medica of Vegetable Origin*

This painting shows the earth, wood, nectarous, and plateau medications used in Tibetan medicine. Earth and mineral medicines have to be detoxified and incinerated before being powdered and used as medication.

Trees, nectars, shrubs grown in hot plains, and herbs should grow in their natural habitat (for example, cool potency plants should grow in a cool climate, and hot potency plants should grow in a hot climate). They should be collected at the right time, detoxified, and stored properly. The duration of potency is discussed here, as are specifications for compounding the ingredients, and the pharmacological techniques to make them easier to ingest and assimilate.

Earth medications include saltpeter, yellow ochre, natron, bitumens, sulphur, vitriol, lichen, and others. Saltpeter helps dissolve kidney, gall bladder, and urinary stones. Yellow ochre helps cure fever of the channels, heals wounds to the five full organs, dries up pus and blood, and heals burns. Sulphur pacifies demonic possession, and dries up pus, blood, and serum. Bitumens aid rejuvenation and alleviate fevers, especially those connected with the stomach, liver, and kidneys.

Wood medication is compounded from roots, tree trunks, branches, bark, sap, leaves, flowers, and fruit. Examples of wood medication are white and red sandalwood from the trunk, myrobalan *(Terminalia chebula)* from the fruit, cinnamon from the bark, frankincense from sap, and birthwort *(Aristolochia)* from the branches.

White sandalwood eliminates heart and lung disease, and alleviates agitated fever. Myrobalan is a panacea and balances the three *nyes-pas.* Cinnamon helps to strengthen the digestive system and the liver, and it pacifies *rlung.* Frankincense subdues demonic influences and acts as an analgesic. Birthwort helps fever of the blood and blood diseases.

Examples of nectarous medication are saffron and nutmeg. Saffron eliminates all diseases connected with the liver, and stops bleeding. Nutmeg subdues *rlung* and eliminates heart disease.

Examples of medication from shrubs grown in hot plains are gentian *(Swertia chirata)* and red bartsia *(Phlogacanthus pubinervius).* Gentian eliminates all diseases connected with the liver and gall bladder, and red bartsia eliminates poisons and fever connected with the blood.

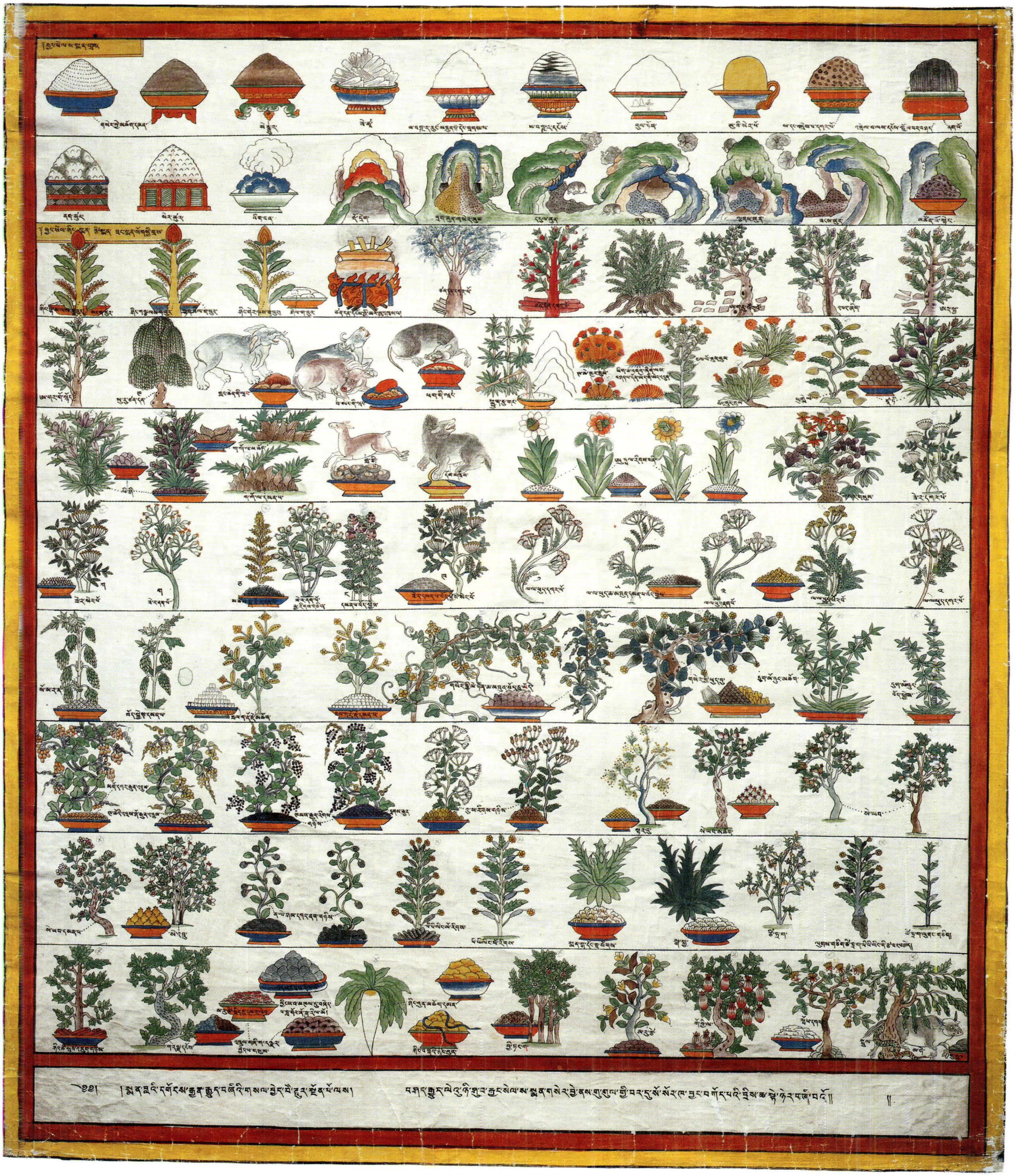

26. *Materia Medica of Vegetable Origin*

Tibet is called Men-Jong, the Land of Medicine; this painting shows the many herbal medications used in Tibetan medicine.

Before the Chinese invaded Tibet in 1950 there were more than three hundred species of medicinal plants that grew in Tibet, and their supply was plentiful. However, when a survey was conducted in 1990 many were found to be extinct, including white sedum, fritillaria, *Codonopsis nervosa,* angelica, and ginseng root. The remaining medicinal plants were also found to be greatly reduced, especially in the Kongpo region of Tibet (east of Lhasa and before Khamdo), and around Lhamo Lhatso, the sacred lake where the birthplace of the Fourteenth Dalai Lama was foreseen. Many Chinese come to stay at the lake for three months, to take a powerful medicinal plant tonic called *yar-tsa-ghun-bu* (summer grass, winter worm). After the invasion of Tibet, the Chinese authorities appropriated and exported hundreds of thousands of kilos of the tonic, as well as fritillaria, wickweed *(Phlomis),* heracleum root, *Codonopsis nervosa,* and other medicinal plants. All of these plants were dug up from the roots with no program of replanting. This has had a very destructive effect on the Tibetan environment and on the future supply of Tibetan herbal medicine.

In this painting are shown herbal medications and their medicinal uses.

Wild rose pacifies *rlung* and eliminates jaundice. Lagotis grass helps to alleviate fevers of the full organs, turbid fever, and rigidity of the thighs caused by *rlung* disorders. Swertia alleviates fevers of the hollow organs, and jaundice. White gentian alleviates sore throat and fevers caused by poisons. Fritillaria heals fractures of the skull and alleviates fevers caused by poisoning. "Blue-thorned" poppy *(Meconopsis horridula/paniculata)* can heal fractured bones, alleviate fevers of the bones, and strengthen cancellate bone. Angelica alleviates fever in the heart, and poisoning. The flowers and fruit of barberries *(Berberis asiatica)* cure diarrhea. Carex alleviates eye diseases and strengthens the eyes; it is also a remedy for wounds to the trunk. Catnip *(Nepeta cataria)* removes albugo from the cornea. Policeman's helmet *(Impatiens)* regulates heavy periods. Tansy *(Tanacetum vulgare)* stops hemorrhages, reduces water retension in the limbs, alleviates kidney disease, and has general rejuvenating properties. Lakeweed *(Polygonum polystachyum)* alleviates serum disorders and edema. Withlow grass *(Dontostemon)* cures meat poisons. Caltrops alleviates water retension, arthritis, and kidney disease. Columbine removes foreign bodies such as an arrowhead, or a dead embryo. Strawberry extracts blood, pus, and serum. Cumin treats eye disease, poison, and fever caused by *rlung* disorder. Larkspur *(Delphinium kamaonense huth)* treats diarrhea.

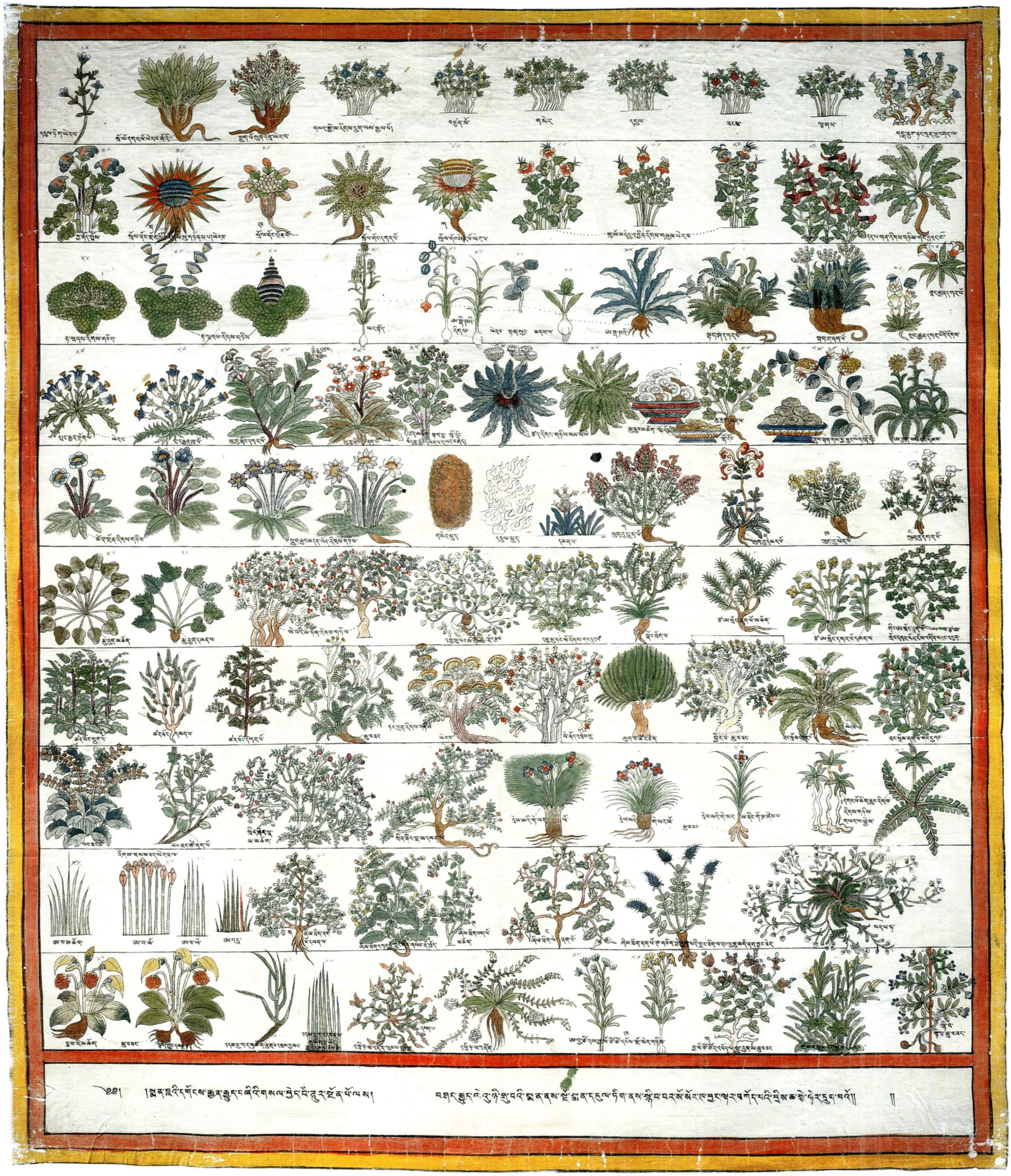

27. Materia Medica of Vegetable and Animal Origin

This description of herbal medications and their medicinal properties is a continuation from the preceding painting (plate 26).

Sweet clover and valerian cure chronic fever and fever caused by poisons. Hogs' fennel *(Angelica)* treats serum and cold kidney disorders, and lumbar problems. Asparagus and Solomon's seal *(Polygonatum)* promote longevity and treat serum. Four-o'clock *(Mirabalis)* root increases male potency, strengthens the kidneys, and dries up serums. Tamarisk and male fern treat meat poisoning and compounded poisoning. Knotgrass *(Polygonum camponulatum)* treats fever of the hollow organs and the small and large intestines. Tibetan lancea strengthens the lungs, and extracts pus from the lungs.

Other plants having medicinal properties are as follows.

Himalayan primrose *(Primula capitata)* cures contagious poisons and chronic fevers. Nodding dragon head *(Draccephalum tanguticum)* alleviates fevers in the stomach, and hepatitis. Marsh mallow *(Malva)* alleviates urine retension, fever of the kidneys, and diarrhea. Shepherd's purse *(Capsella bursa pastoris)* cures vomiting. Orchid is a tonic and it increases sperm count. Pennycress treats coughing and kidney infections. Spurge *(Euphorbia)* treats both hot and cold diseases, and is used as an emetic. Rhubarb cleanses *bad-kan* and fever caused by poison, and fever of the hollow organs. Burrweed *(Xanthium strumarium)* alleviates contagious poison, kidney infection, and fever caused by trauma. Indian madder *(Rubia cordifolia)* treats pulmonary and kidney diseases.

In the Tibetan medical texts various kinds of animal products are mentioned, but few are used. As Buddhists, Tibetans try to avoid killing other living beings.

Fish strengthens the eyesight and appetite, heals wounds, dissolves tumors, and strengthens the digestive system. Peacock flesh treats jaundice, poisoning, and demonic possession. Sheep's brain treats vertigo. Goat's brain heals tendons and ligaments. Goat's liver is used as a tonic for the eyes. Otter's liver treats urine retention. Goat's heart treats worms. Rabbit's heart treats angina, madness, and demonic possession. Sheep's bone treats *rlung* disorders. Pig's bone alleviates stomach ulcers. Musk treats worms, inflammation, poisoning, and kidney disorders. Boar treats contagious poisoning, and fever of the liver and hollow organs. Pig's fat treats skin diseases, gathers poisons together, and promotes hair growth. Snake skin treats lucoderma (a type of skin disease) and eczema. Wild yak's horn dissolves tumors and improves body heat.

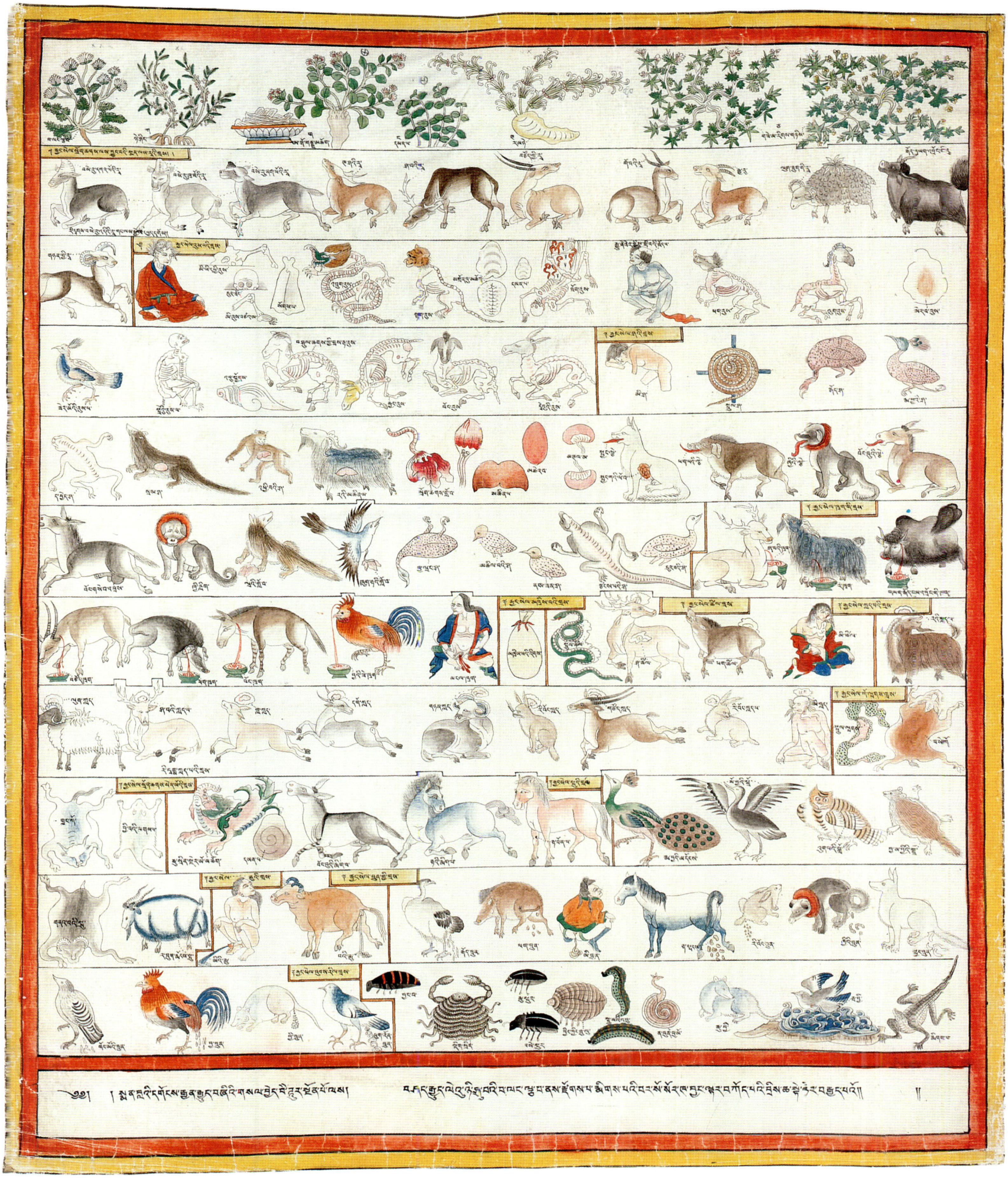

28. *Sundry Painting: Examining the Tongue; The Nine Particular Therapeutic Principles; The Making of Medicine; Herbal Remedies; Oil Therapy*

The tongue of a patient with a *rlung* disorder is reddish, dry, and coarse in texture; with a *mkhris-pa* disorder it is light yellow, with a thick coating; with a *bad-kan* disorder it is pale, with a smooth and moist texture. The tongue of a dying patient is black, dry in the middle, and it cannot be extended; there is also loss of voice.

There are nine methods of dealing with diseases. When the physician needs to confirm a diagnosis he can, for example, give the patient a decoction of gentian; if the patient responds positively there is a *mkhris-pa* disorder. Throughout this process the physician should be as cautious as a cat. Once the physician has confidence in the diagnosis he can explain the causes, symptoms, and treatment of the disease to the patient, as if hoisting a banner on the top of a mountain.

Some diseases require the physician to prescribe a medicine to bring the disease out; it can then be treated with medication to eradicate it. This method is compared to taming a wild horse and putting it in a stable.

If the patient comes to the physician after having previously seen another doctor, the physician will have to ascertain whether the previous doctor prescribed the correct medication at an appropriate dosage. The physician must investigate the disease like a gull catching fish. If the disease is very serious, the physician must act quickly and treat it by prescribing the four water therapies: fasting by taking only water and no solid food; cooling the body by taking cold baths; taking medicine such as a camphor decoction; and undergoing minor surgery such as bloodletting. This situation is compared to meeting your enemy in a narrow lane, where there is no retreat or escape. Minor diseases are treated gradually, with advice on diet and behavior; prescribing medicine; and performing surgery. This method is compared to slowly ascending a staircase one step at a time. Individual diseases can be treated separately, without disturbing the other humors. This is compared to a warrior destroying an enemy on the spot. Multiple or combined diseases, such as combinations of humoral disorders, should be treated with equanimity, like a chieftan making peace between two warring parties.

It is very important to consider the patient's bodily constitution, strength, age, metabolic rate, and seasonal factors in order to prescribe the right medication or perform the right kind of surgery. Otherwise prescriptions can be as foolish as putting the load of a *dzo* on the back of a sheep.

Tibetan medications are prepared as decoctions, powders, pills, medicinal pastes, medicinal butters, medicinal ashes, concentrated decoctions, medicinal wines, gem medicines, and herbal compounds. The most popular medicines today are pills.

Before performing the external therapies (purgatives, emetics, nasal medications, and mild and strong enemas), the physician performs oil therapy, using vegetable oils, melted butter, bone marrow, and/or animal fats. The oil can be massaged on the body and head, or taken internally through the mouth or rectum. Oil therapy is advisable for older people, people suffering from severe stress and tension, malnutrition, impotency, or disorders of a *rlung* nature.

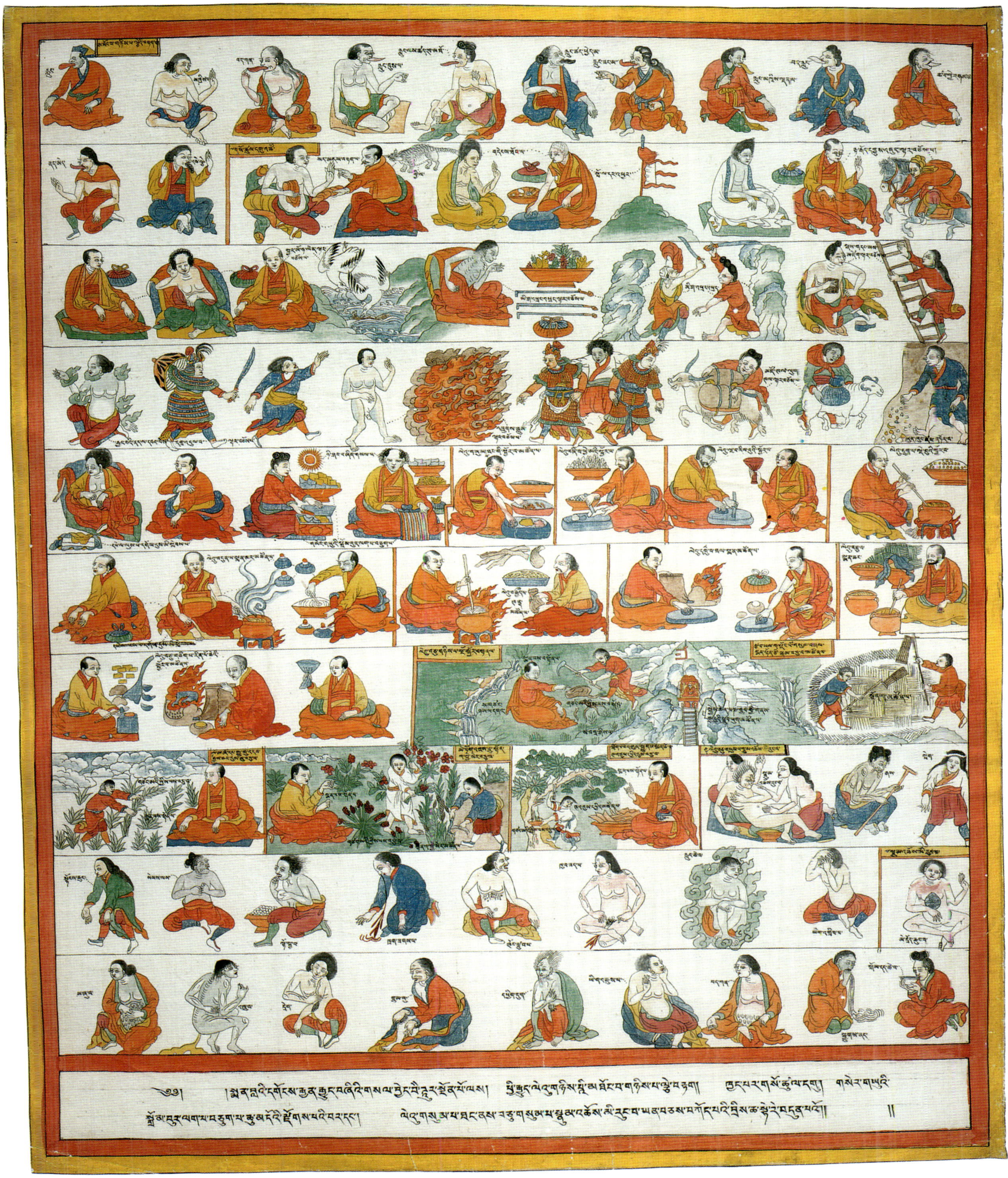

29. *Ritual Preparation of Rejuvenation Elixirs*

The majority of this painting deals with the generation of the Lesser Elixir of Rejuvenation through visualizations of the light-ray emanations from the celestial palace of medicine in the center. The physician (the man seated to the left of the palace) is instructed to visualize himself as a meditational deity as he gathers the rejuvenation elixirs from the realms of gods, antigods, humans, animals, tormented spirits, and the hell realm (all shown below the palace). Major Buddhas, boddhisattvas, and goddesses, whose compassion and spirituality are absorbed into the elixirs, are pictured at the top of the painting.

In the lower part of the painting is a panel showing the ideal surroundings to enhance sexual pleasure and, therefore, fertility. It is important to choose the right place to make love, and to create the right mood. The environment should be tranquil, surrounded by waterfalls, flowers, and natural sounds, and it should have a relaxed atmosphere. For sexual pleasure, the main factor is a virile man —otherwise even if he were surrounded by a hundred beautiful women it would still be no good. The woman should be young, pretty, clean, sweet spoken and well mannered, wearing nice clothes and jewels. Physical behavior should include kissing, embracing, touching, good conversation, massaging, and relaxation. The diet should be one of molasses, honey, milk, and meat broth—generally sweet foods to increase the generative fluid.

The painting of the Greater Elixir of Rejuvenation (painting 52; not in this volume) describes how a program of rejuvenation can prolong life; enhance memory, intelligence, and youth; strengthen the body and the senses; and increase vigor. The environment for rejuvenation should be clean, unpolluted, and natural. There should be waterfalls, greenery, no disruptions, and it should be quiet. The person to be rejuvenated should not be too old, they should avoid sexual intercourse and be free from stress. They should avoid too much sun and heat, and they should avoid raw, sour, stale, and salty foods. They should be rejuvenated on an auspicious day, and they should pray and cleanse themselves.

Rejuvenation through taking compounded medications can be followed as a part-time or full-time program.

For the full-time rejuvenation program, you should eat oily and warm potency food, and have fomentation administered. For cleansing the system, you should then take an herbal preparation of myrobalan *(Terminalia chebula)*, embelic myrobalan, rock salt, long pepper *(Piper longum)*, white sweet flag *(Acorus calamus)*, dry ginger, tumeric, false black pepper *(Embelia ribes)*, and molasses. This preparation will purge the system, which is very important before rejuvenation.

Substances used in rejuvenation are the five essences and the four nectars. The five essences include essence of soil (iron bitumens, which rejuvenate the muscle tissue), essence of minerals (calcite, which rejuvenates the bones), essence of wood (molasses, which gives vigor), essence of flowers (honey, which rejuvenates the skin), and essence of grass (butter, which rejuvenates the reproductive fluid).

The four nectars are juniper berries, rhododendron flower, ephedra, and tansy *(Tanacetum vulgare)*.

If you can combine all nine ingredients (five essences and four nectars) and use them, all signs of aging will disappear and your body will become as young as that of a sixteen-year-old. You will have the prowess of a lion, strength of an elephant, complexion of a peacock, speed of a stallion, and your lifespan will be like the sun and moon. Also beneficial are long-life prayers to Tara and Amitabha.

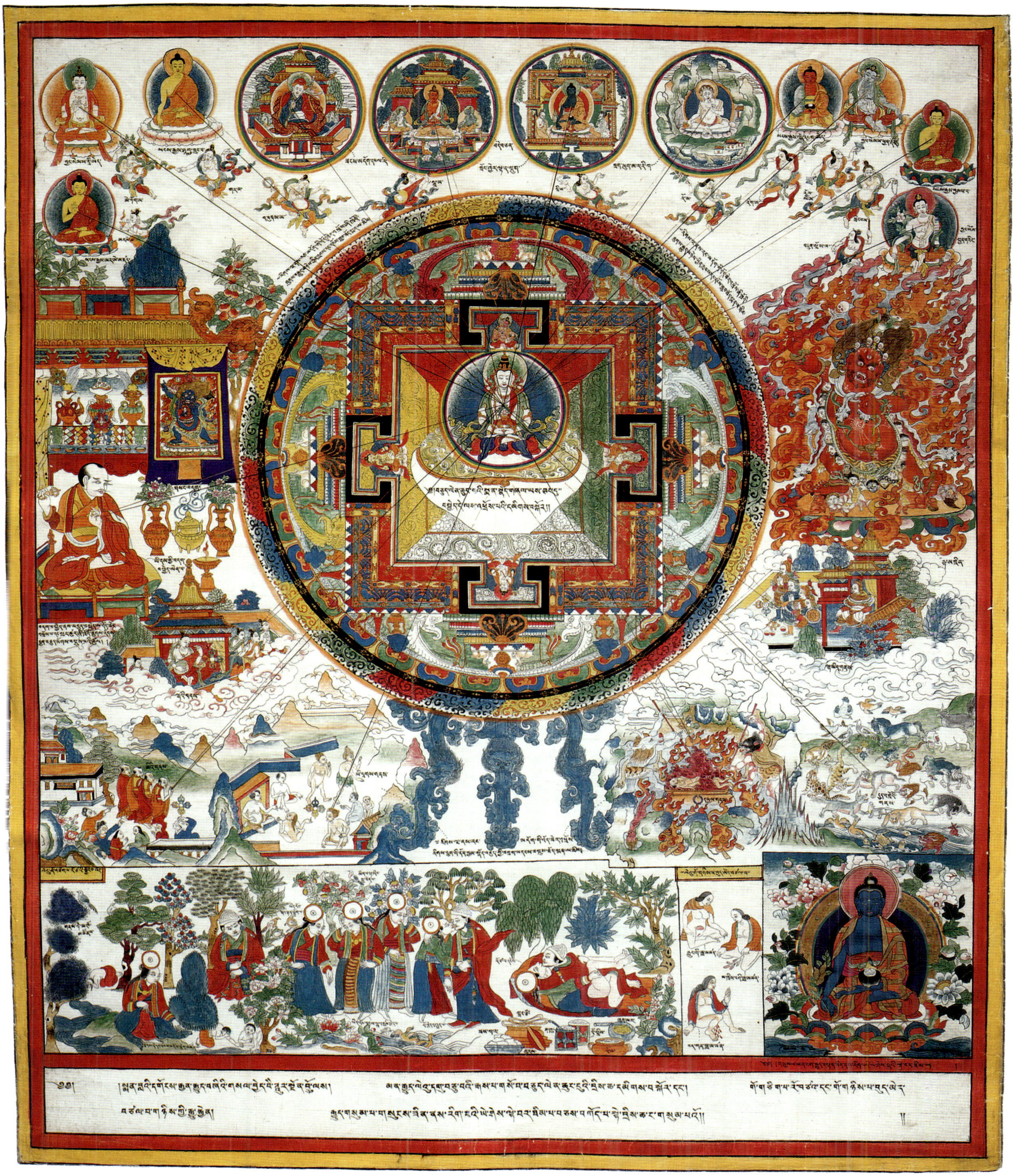

30. *Cleansing Therapies*

This painting and the following painting depict the five external therapeutic techniques in Tibetan medicine: purgatives, emetics, nasal medication, mild enema, and strong enema.

Purgatives are mainly used for cleansing *mkhris-pa.* They are beneficial for contagious, disturbed, unripened, and fully developed fevers. They are also used to alleviate poisons, fevers of the hollow organs, tumors, edema, leprosy, gout, arthritis, worms, chronic wounds, and so on. Purgatives are not beneficial for people with weak bodily constitutions, older people, those suffering from demonic possession, pregnant women, those suffering from a *rlung* disorder, or people with diseases of the rectum. Purgatives are also not suitable if a foreign body such as a bullet or an arrowhead is in the system.

The herbal ingredients used for purgatives are a "beak-shaped" myrobalan *(Terminalia chebula),* croton, madar grass *(Caltropis gigantea),* and spurge *(Euphorbia).* Before being used the individual ingredients are detoxified and then powdered.

Emetics are used for the cleansing of excess *bad-kan* from the system. They are used to treat indigestion, tumors, loss of appetite, worms, gastritis, and all diseases connected with the digestive system. They are not beneficial for people with weak bodily constitutions, those with *rlung* disorders, urine retention, cataracts, hemorrhoids, meat poisoning, or children under sixteen and adults over seventy. The herbal ingredients used for emetics are mountain sorrel, thistle, spurge *(Euphorbia),* sweet flag *(Acorus calamus),* rock salt, and long pepper *(Piper longum).* These ingredients are used as a base, and additional ingredients are then added according to the individual nature of the disease.

Gentle nasal medication is beneficial for diseases related to the head, because the nose is like a door to the brain. Nasal medication is not an effective treatment for wounds, nor is it appropriate for someone who has consumed too much alcohol or oil, or someone who has just suffered an epidermic fever. Gentle nasal medications are a combination of saffron, crystal sugar, and melted butter. They will relieve headaches caused by *rlung* and blood disorders.

Strong nasal medication is not beneficial for vertigo, dizziness due to *rlung* disorders, bleeding and pus discharge from the gums, or blurry eyes. It is beneficial for chronic catarrh of the nasal cavities, bloodshot eyes, a swollen face caused by a serum disorder, and cranial fractures. Strong nasal medications are a combination of strawberries, sea salt, sweet flag *(Acorus calamus),* costus *(Sanssurea lappa),* and licorice.

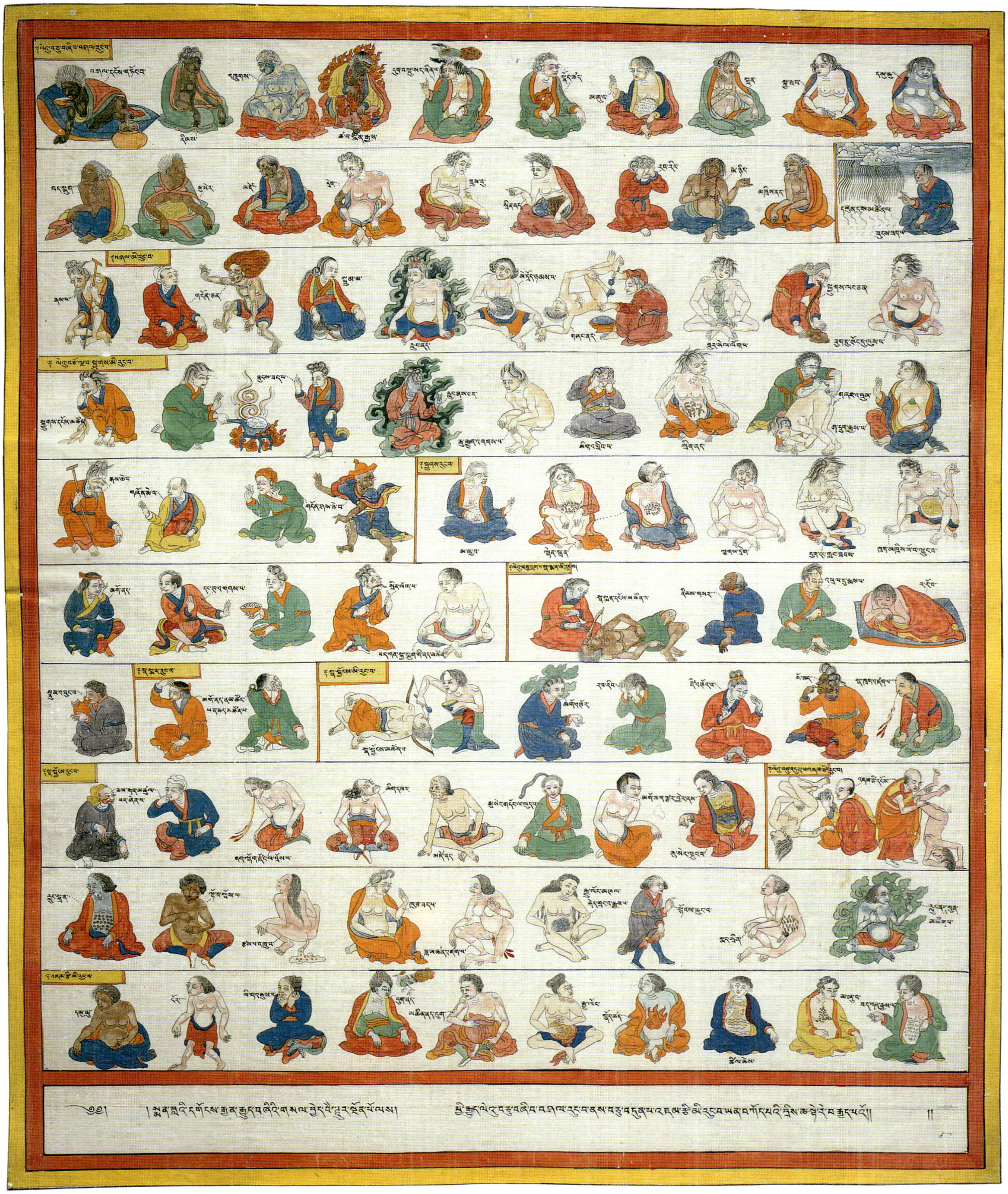

31. *Cleansing and Bloodletting Therapies*

This painting is a continuation from the preceding painting (plate 30). Bloodletting is also illustrated in plate 33. Indications and contraindications for various cleansing therapies are illustrated.

Mild enemas are beneficial for tumors caused by *rlung* disorders, flatulence, diarrhea, deficiency of sperm count, and heavy periods. They are also used to treat cold diseases related to the small intestine, large intestine, kidneys, and lumbar region. Mild enemas are unsuitable for chronic edema, loss of appetite, poisons, liver disorders, obesity, indigestion, or excessive *bad-kan.*

Strong enemas can be used to treat constipation, abdominal spasms, urine retention, a bloated stomach, worms, newly developed tumors, and chronic epidermic fever. They are particularly effective for virulent diseases. They are unsuitable for prolapse of the rectum, chronic diarrhea, spermatorrhea, and newly developed fevers.

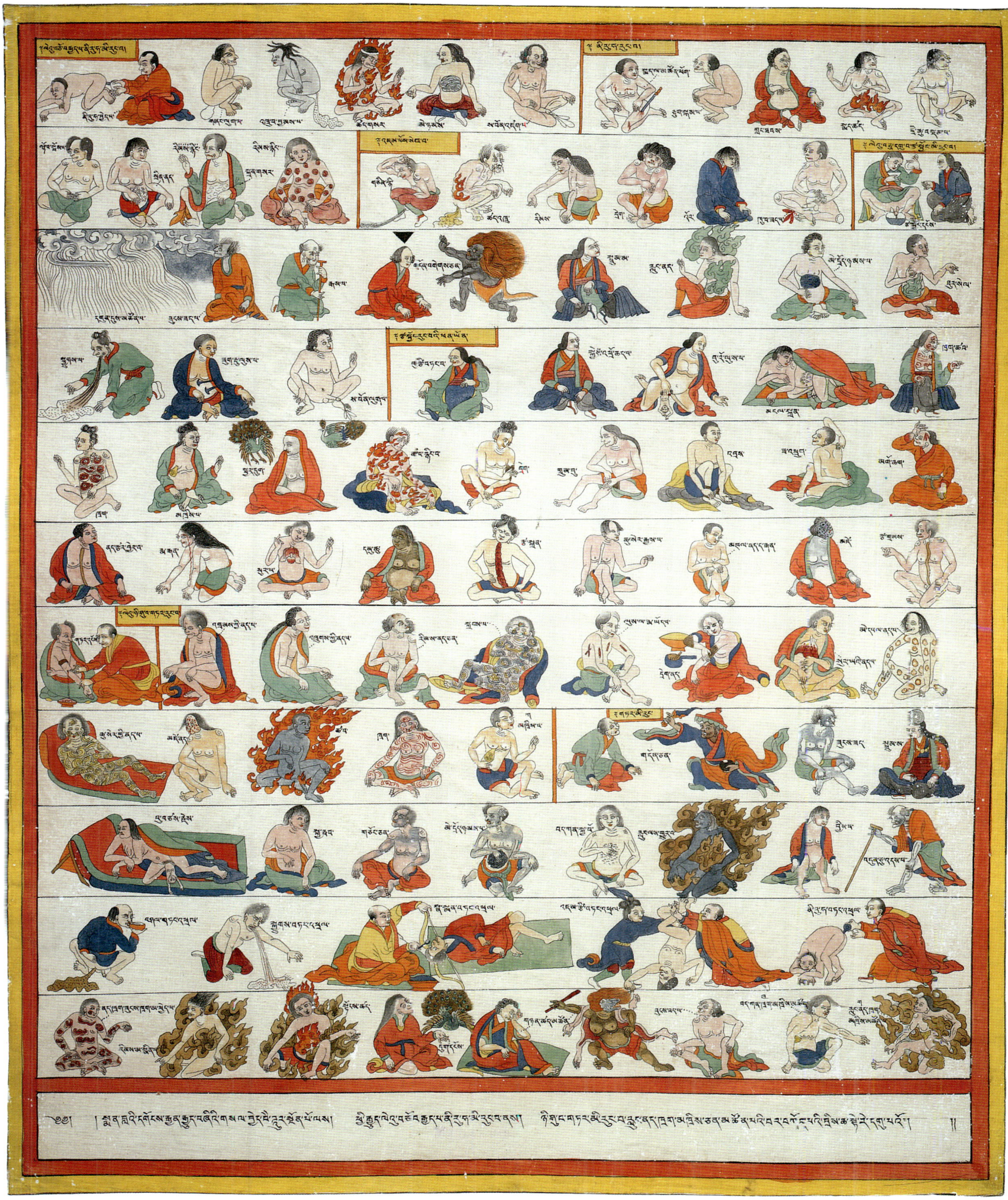

32. Medical Instruments

This painting shows the surgical instruments used in performing therapy in Tibetan medicine.

There are three categories of performing therapy: mild, rough, and rigorous. Mild therapy involves compresses, fomentation, and massage. Rough therapy includes bloodletting, moxibustion, and minor surgery. Rigorous therapies consist of incision, excision, scraping, and extraction.

Surgical instruments include probes, forceps, lancets, stylets, and other auxiliary instruments.

Probes are used for exploring cranial bone fractures, and excision of hemorrhoids. Probing instruments are round, thin, and smoothly polished for cranial exploration. For hemorrhoids there are a series of tubular probes with lateral openings for examination and incision.

Forceps include lion-mouth forceps, kite-beaked forceps, and crow-beaked forceps. They are used for extracting foreign bodies from muscle tissues and ligaments.

Lancets are used mainly for incision into muscle tissue and for puncturing vessels to cause bleeding. They include the sparrow-feather-shaped lancet, the axe-shaped lancet, the curved lancet (which is six finger-widths in length), and the sickle-shaped lancet used to incise tongue swellings.

Stylets are used to make punctures to release fluids or vapors from various parts of the body. They include hollow surgical stylets, the frog-shaped stylet, and the reed-nib-shaped stylet.

Auxiliary instruments include two medical saws, a sharp medical knife, trephine and uterine stylets, snake-head-shaped stylets, and catheter instruments. All are made from the finest iron, copper, and gold, and are well polished. They come in different shapes and lengths.

Very few of these are used, as in Tibetan medicine performing surgery is a last resort when treating a patient.

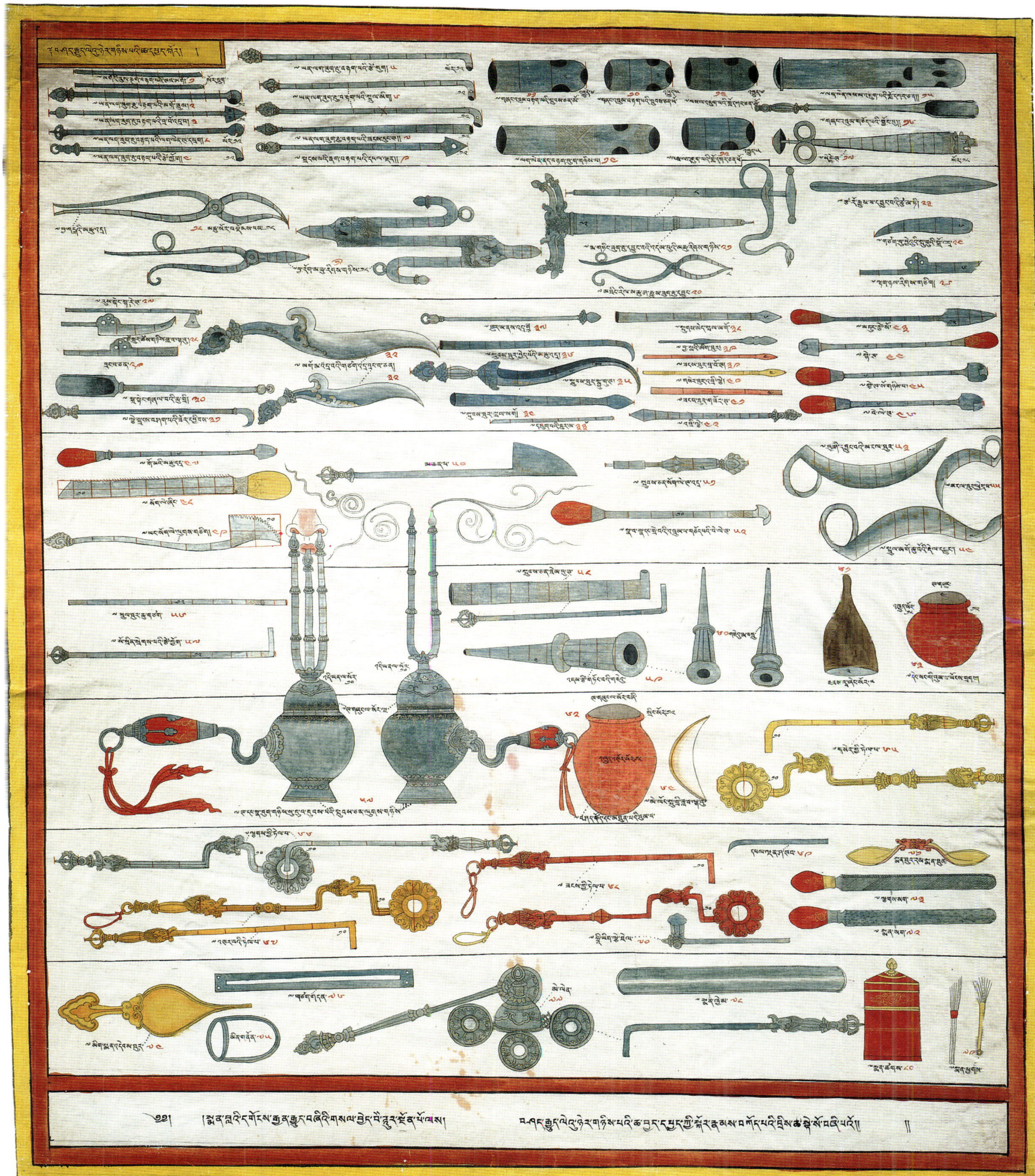

33. *Bloodletting and Moxibustion*

This painting shows the bloodletting points in the human body, and outlines the indications for moxibustion.

In Tibetan medicine bloodletting is considered to be one of the most effective therapeutic techniques. It is very important, however, that it is performed by an experienced physician—otherwise it might have extremely adverse effects.

The instrument used in bloodletting is a lancet shaped like a sparrow's feather, curved like a crescent moon, and six finger-widths in length. Or it should be a "supine-shaped" lancet. The blade should be sharp enough to shave hair and it should be made by the most skilled blacksmith, using the best refined iron available.

Bloodletting is suitable for *mkhris-pa* diseases and blood disorders such as leprosy, gout, ringworm, erysipelas, serum disorders, body wounds, and contagious fevers. It is not suitable for pregnancy, postnatal conditions, edema, consumption, lack of digestive heat, people with weak bodily constitutions, children under sixteen, adults over seventy, or people with *rlung* and *bad-kan* disorders.

Three or five days before the bloodletting is performed, the patient should take a decoction made from three different types of myrobalan, moonseed *(Menispermum canadense)*, elecompane *(Inula helenium)*, and birthwort *(Aristolochia)* to separate the pure and impure blood. On the day of bloodletting the patient should keep warm and stay in the sun to improve blood circulation. The blood vessels in the part of the body where the bloodletting is going to be performed should then be tightened for easy incision.

Bloodletting purifies the body system, strengthens channels, reduces pain and swelling, and dries up pus. If the patient is thin it can help him gain weight, and if he is too fat it can help him lose weight.

The best time to collect the flowers used in moxibustion (gerbera) is in the autumn. They should be thoroughly dried and made into the shape of a small cone so that it can be easily attached to the precise moxibustion points.

Moxibustion is performed mainly for *rlung* and *bad-kan* disorders such as indigestion, lack of digestive heat, edema, tumors, madness, dementia, and channel disorders. It is not good when performed directly on the five sense organs or the genitalia. Moxibustion can dry up serum, improve body temperature, help digestion, improve body heat, and enhance memory. Moxibustion is not an effective treatment for *mkhris-pa* and blood disorders.

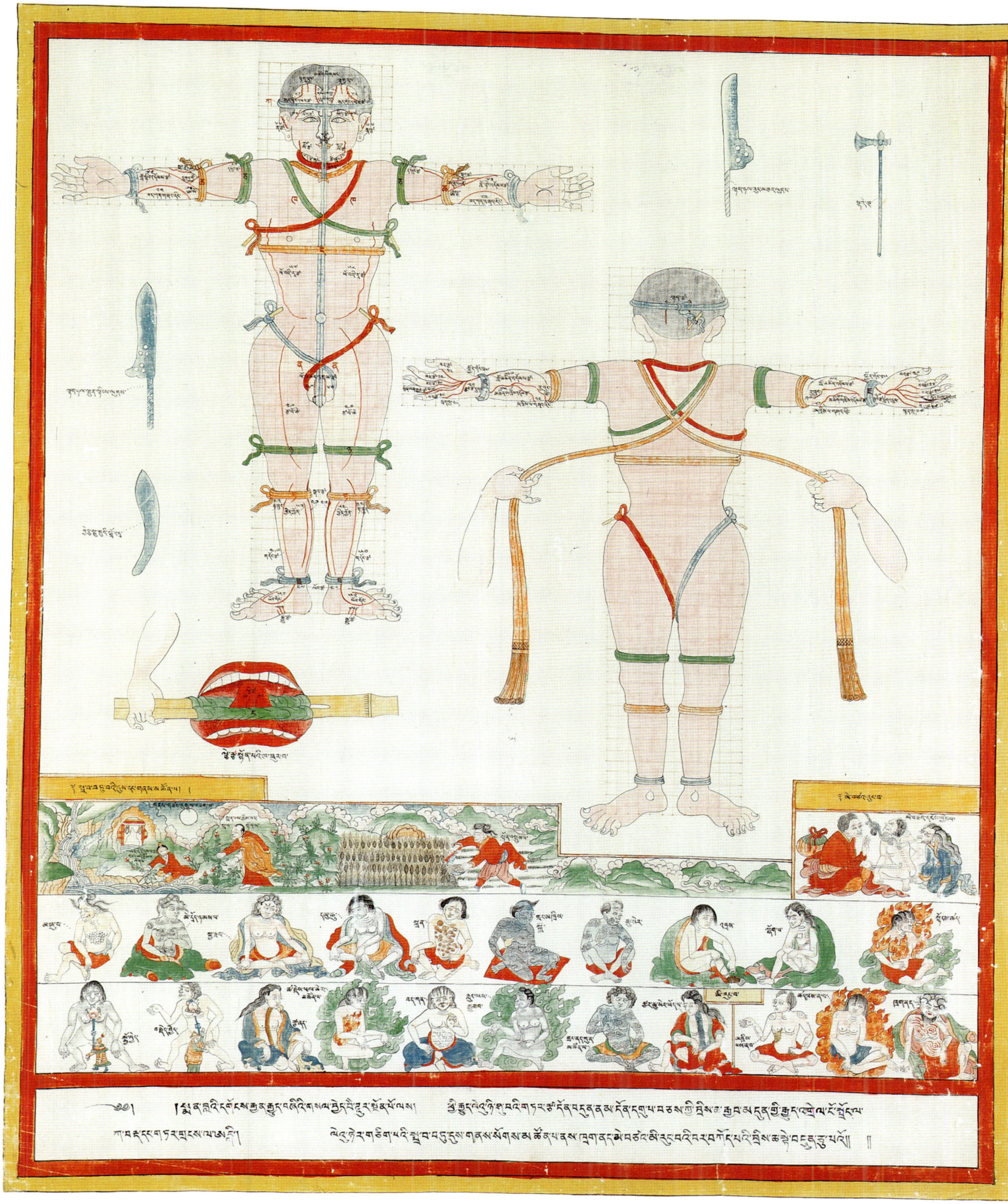

34. Sundry Painting: Compresses; Fomentation; Ointments; Minor Surgery

External therapies such as bloodletting, moxibustion, and minor surgery are discussed in the descriptions of plates 32 and 33. The points for these therapies are pictured in plates 35 and 36. This painting describes compresses, fomentation, and ointments used in Tibetan medicine.

Compresses (dealt with in the first two rows) are the most effective painkillers in Tibetan medicine. There are eleven cold compresses and nineteen hot compresses. Cold compresses include cold pebbles, and water collected beneath the stars. Cold river pebbles treat imbalances of the blood and *mkhris-pa,* and abdominal spasms due to fever. Black mud collected beneath the stars is used to stop nasal bleeding. Hot compresses include applying heated river pebbles and heated salt wrapped in cloth; these treat indigestion, and abdominal and colon spasms. Compresses are especially beneficial for *bad-kan* and *rlung* disorders, indigestion, serum disorders, abdominal and colon spasms, coagulation of the blood, and pain caused by fever. They are unsuitable for edema, advanced jaundice, leprosy, poisoning, and so on.

The next two sections deal with wrapping fomentations, combinations of medicinal ingredients such as rhododendron, juniper, ephedra, tamarisk, and tansy *(Tanacetum vulgare),* which are mixed with water and boiled. The patient is then placed in a big bathtub to soak for a long time; this helps people suffering from paralysis or from a slipped disc. It will also ease the muscles, nerves, ligaments, and tendons. Fomentation is beneficial for lameness, muscular spasms, stiffness, gynecological diseases, spinal deformities, serum disorders of muscle and bone tissue, chronic wounds, and all problems related to *rlung* disorders. It is not suitable for people with weak bodily constitutions, or for the treatment of edema, loss of appetite, or fully developed fevers. Fomentation is not advisable on the eyes, cheeks, big toes, elbows that are affected by gout, the penis, stomach, or any area around the heart. Fomentation is like a medicated sauna; the infused steam helps to draw all serum and impurities from the body pores. It reduces *rlung,* reduces swelling, and after fomentation a thin person will gain weight.

Ointments, discussed in the following two sections, consist of oils and medicinal paste applications. For oil application, first the oil is applied, massaged, and then wiped from the skin with flour. It will help to clear deposits of fats (cellulite) and to clear the channels. To enhance the memory, oil can be applied and massaged with melted butter; to treat eczema, oil is applied with black sulphur mixed with pork fat; to help insomnia, oil is applied with musk and melted butter all over the body and the head.

Medicinal pastes can be made with soot, tumeric, barberries *(Berberis asiatica),* costus *(Sanssurea lappa),* kurchee *(Holarrhena antidysenterica)* and buttermilk. Medicinal pastes treat pimples and blemishes. Pastes of snake skin and pork fat treat lucoderma.

Ointments are beneficial for rough skin, deficiency of blood and reproductive fluids, weak bodily constitutions, old age, grief, mental stress, insomnia, exhaustion, retinitis pigmentosa and *rlung* disorders. They are not suitable for indigestion, gemstone poisoning, loss of appetite, edema, or brown *bad-kan* disorders.

The last two sections of the painting describe indications and contraindications for minor surgery.

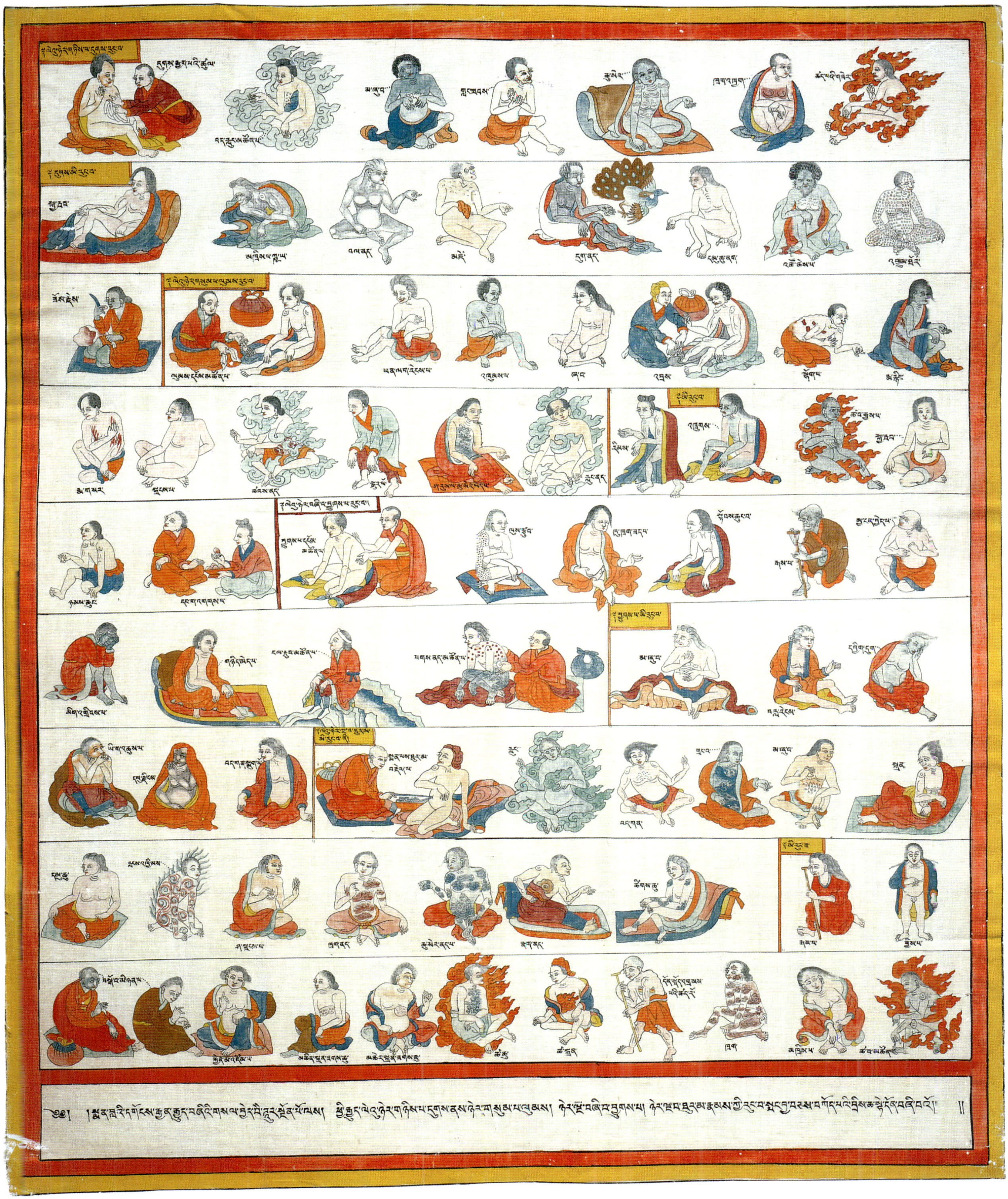

35. The Points for Bloodletting, Moxibustion, and Minor Surgery: Front View

In Tibetan medicine there are seventy-seven bloodletting points: twenty-one points in the head and neck, thirty-four in the arms, eighteen in the legs, two in the stomach, and two in the penis.

Impure blood is thin, yellowish, and full of mucus and pus. When bloodletting is performed the blood flows very forcefully. If the blood is dark black and lines are visible it means that the patient needs an herbal decoction to separate the pure and impure blood before further bloodletting. If the blood is black, coarse, and its foam is red, it means that the patient has a *rlung* disorder. If the blood is yellowish, thin, and has a pus odor, it means that the patient has a *mkhris-pa* disorder. If the blood is light, red, thick, and smooth, it is a *bad-kan* disorder. If the blood is as red as red lac (a medicinal soil), it means that it is good blood—if this blood is produced during bloodletting the procedure must be stopped and not a drop should be wasted as this blood sustains our life.

The anterior view shows bloodletting points such as the anterior fontanel, vessels of the eyes, tip of the nose, vessels of the tongue, middle of the lower lip, mediocephalic veins, jugular vein, superficial temporal, tibial veins, cephalic veins, radial veins, great saphenous vein, and blood vessels of the small intestine.

In Tibetan medicine there are seventy-one points for placing moxa: twenty on the posterior side of the body, twenty-two on the anterior side of the body, and twenty-nine on the head and limbs.

The main anterior moxibustion points are as follows. Moxa placed on the crown of the head and anterior fontanel points treats vertigo and *rlung* disorders. Moxa placed on the nape treats mental disorders. Moxa placed on the sternum point treats madness and depression. Moxa placed one inch below the xiphoid point (the tumor point) treats stomach tumors. One inch below the navel, to the left, center, and right, are the upper intestine points, and one inch below these to the left, center, and right are the lower intestine points. Moxa placed on all these points treats diarrhea caused by the disturbance of *rlung.* Moxa placed on the suprasternal point treats hiccups, blockages of the throat, and eases dislocation of the heart. Moxa placed on the big toes points treats stiffness of the neck, and swollen testicles. Moxa placed on the middle of the left and right shoulder points treats nose bleeding.

Minor surgery is mainly performed to drain fluids, pus, and impure blood from the five full organs and six hollow organs.

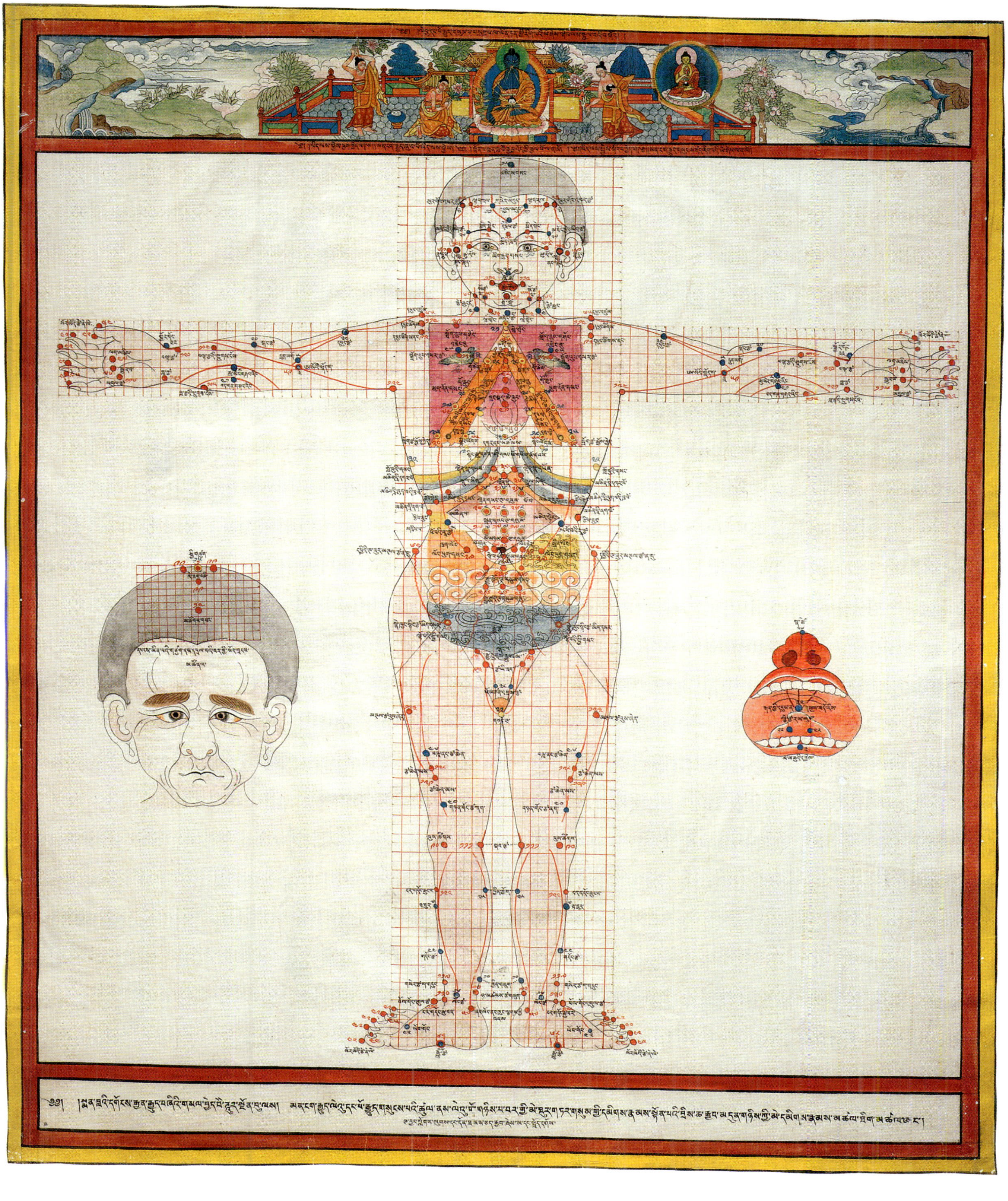

36. The Points for Bloodletting, Moxibustion, and Minor Surgery: Back View

Important posterior bloodletting points are the crown of the head, posterior fontanels, pinna, basilic vein, median antebrachial, and so on.

If the disease is connected with the upper part of the body, blood is let from the jugular and radial veins. If the disease is connected with the middle part of the body, blood is let from the mediocephalic and basilic veins. If the disease is connected with the lower part of the body, blood is let from the saphenous and tibial veins.

In the Tibetan medical system the sixth vertebra from the top of the spinal cord according to Western medicine is counted as the first vertebra—the moxa points listed here follow the vertebrae according to the Tibetan system.

This first vertebra is a *rlung* point: moxa placed here will help mental disorders and loss of speech. The second vertebra is a *mkhris-pa* point: moxa placed on this point will help cold *mkhris-pa.* The third vertebra is a *bad-kan* point: moxa placed here helps pulmonary and heart diseases, and headaches caused by cold *mkhris-pa.* The fourth and fifth vertebrae are for the lungs: moxa placed on these will help pulmonary diseases related to *rlung* and *bad-kan* disorders. The sixth and seventh vertebrae are the life channel and heart points: moxa placed on these points will help relieve madness, insomnia, palpitation, heart diseases, and forgetfulness. The eighth vertebra is the diaphragm point and the ninth vertebra is the liver point: moxa placed on these points will help eructation, vomiting, blockage of the diaphragm, liver tumors, and will help strengthen the liver.

The tenth vertebra is the gall bladder point: moxa placed here treats indigestion, yellow eyes jaundice, gallstones, loss of appetite, constant headaches, and lack of digestive heat. The eleventh vertebra is the spleen point: moxa placed here eliminates gas formation, heaviness in the body, and heavy sleep. The twelfth vertebra is the stomach point: moxa placed here treats lack of digestive heat, stomach tumors, and chronic diarrhea. The thirteenth vertebra is the reproductive organs point: moxa placed here treats premature ejaculation, heavy periods, constipation, and tumors of the uterus. The fourteenth vertebra is the kidney point: moxa placed here helps all kidney diseases. The fifteenth vertebra is the common point for the five full and six hollow organs: moxa placed here helps all cold diseases connected with these organs. The sixteenth vertebra is the large intestine point: moxa placed here treats tumors in the large intestine, flatulence, hemorrhoids, urine retention, and urine infection. The seventeenth vertebra is the intestine point: moxa placed here will help treat small intestine tumors, chronic mucus, and diarrhea. The eighteenth vertebra is the urinary bladder point: moxa placed here treats urinary stones, urine retention, and frequency of urine. The nineteenth vertebra is the reproductive fluids point: moxa placed here helps treat premature ejaculation and impotence. The twentieth vertebra is the downward-cleansing *rlung* point: moxa placed here treats incontinence of the bowels, constipation, and mucus diarrhea.

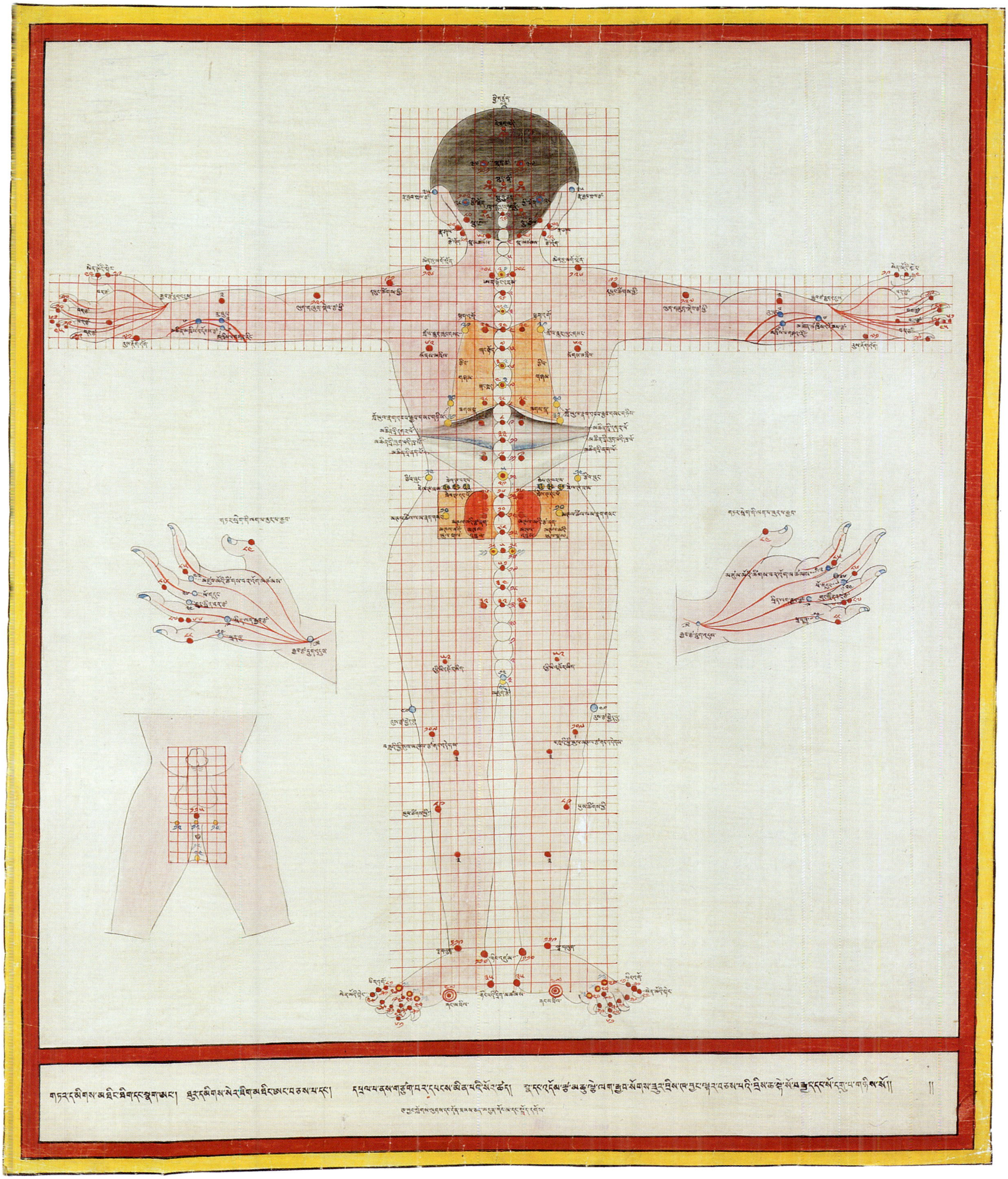

37. Humoral Disorders; Impaired Digestion; Tumors

The primary and secondary causes of *rlung* disturbance are desire (represented by the first image of a bird), excessive eating of light and bitter foods, too much sex, heavy bleeding, chronic diarrhea and vomiting, irregular sleep, mental stress, not eating at the right times, and performing physical and mental activities on an empty stomach.

There are sixty-three types of *rlung*. For example, eight are related to neurological disorders: rigidity, retraction, atrophy, distension, lameness, acute pain, madness, and fainting.

Treatment of *rlung* disorders includes advising the patient to eat more oily and nutritious food, and to sit in dark, quiet, and warm places surrounded by friends and lovers. Medication is a combination of the following medicines: Agar 35, Agar 15, Agar 31, and Asafoedita 25.

The primary and secondary causes of *mkhris-pa* disturbances are hatred and anger (represented by the snake in the third row), excessive eating of hot potency and sour food, injuries caused to the liver and gall bladder, too strenuous physical activity. There are forty-seven types of *mkhris-pa,* divided into yellow skin *mkhris-pa,* yellow eyes *mkhris-pa,* hot *mkhris-pa,* cold *mkhris-pa,* and black *mkhris-pa.*

Yellow skin *mkhris-pa* symptoms are heaviness in the body, uncontrollable sleep, tiredness, a bitter taste in the mouth, and seeing white objects as yellow. The symptoms are worse at noon and better in the early morning. Yellow eyes *mkhris-pa* symptoms are yellowing of the sclera and nails, excess sweating, pain in the eye sockets, loss of appetite, thirst, nausea, and seeing everything as red and blue. Hot *mkhris-pa* symptoms are thirst, a bitter taste, itchiness, lack of sleep, and very yellow stools and urine. Cold *mkhris-pa* symptoms are white stools because of a lack of digestive heat. Black *mkhris-pa* symptoms are advanced jaundice: the skin becomes black, there is loss of hair on the head and eyebrows, weight loss, tiredness, and yellowing of the nails. Jaundice spreads to the whole body and at this time there is no hope for treatment—otherwise Tibetan medicine is very successful in treating jaundice and hepatitis.

Treatment for *mkhris-pa* disorders involves advising less greasy foods and a light diet. Medications prescribed are a combination of gentian, kurchee *(Holarrhena antidysenterica),* monkshood *(Aconitum naviculare/Heterophyllum wall),* sow thistle *(Sonchus),* spleenwort *(Chrysosplenium),* and swertia, among others.

The primary and secondary causes of *bad-kan* disturbance are delusion (represented by the pig in the fifth row), and excessive eating of oily, bitter, heavy, sweet, and cooling foods. Improper conduct such as sleeping in the daytime, getting no exercise, or exposure to the cold can disturb *bad-kan.* There are forty-one types of *bad-kan,* and they are connected with lack of digestive heat: difficulty swallowing, malabsorption, indigestion, anorexia, and so on.

Treatment involves advising a warm diet of cooked foods, drinking lots of hot water, getting plenty of exercise, and keeping warm. Medications prescribed are a combination of quince, elecompane *(Inula helenium),* coriander, sea buckthorn *(Hippophae rhamnoids),* poppy, pomegranate, galangal *(Kaempferia galangala),* embelic myrobalan, and calcite, among others.

Indigestion is caused by eating raw, uncooked foods, eating irregularly, or eating without having properly digested previous food. Foods will not be digested and absorbed by the body; they will turn into mucus, block the channels, and disrupt the whole system. This leads to tumors in the five full and six hollow organs.

It is very important to eat sensibly, at the right time, and in the right quantity.

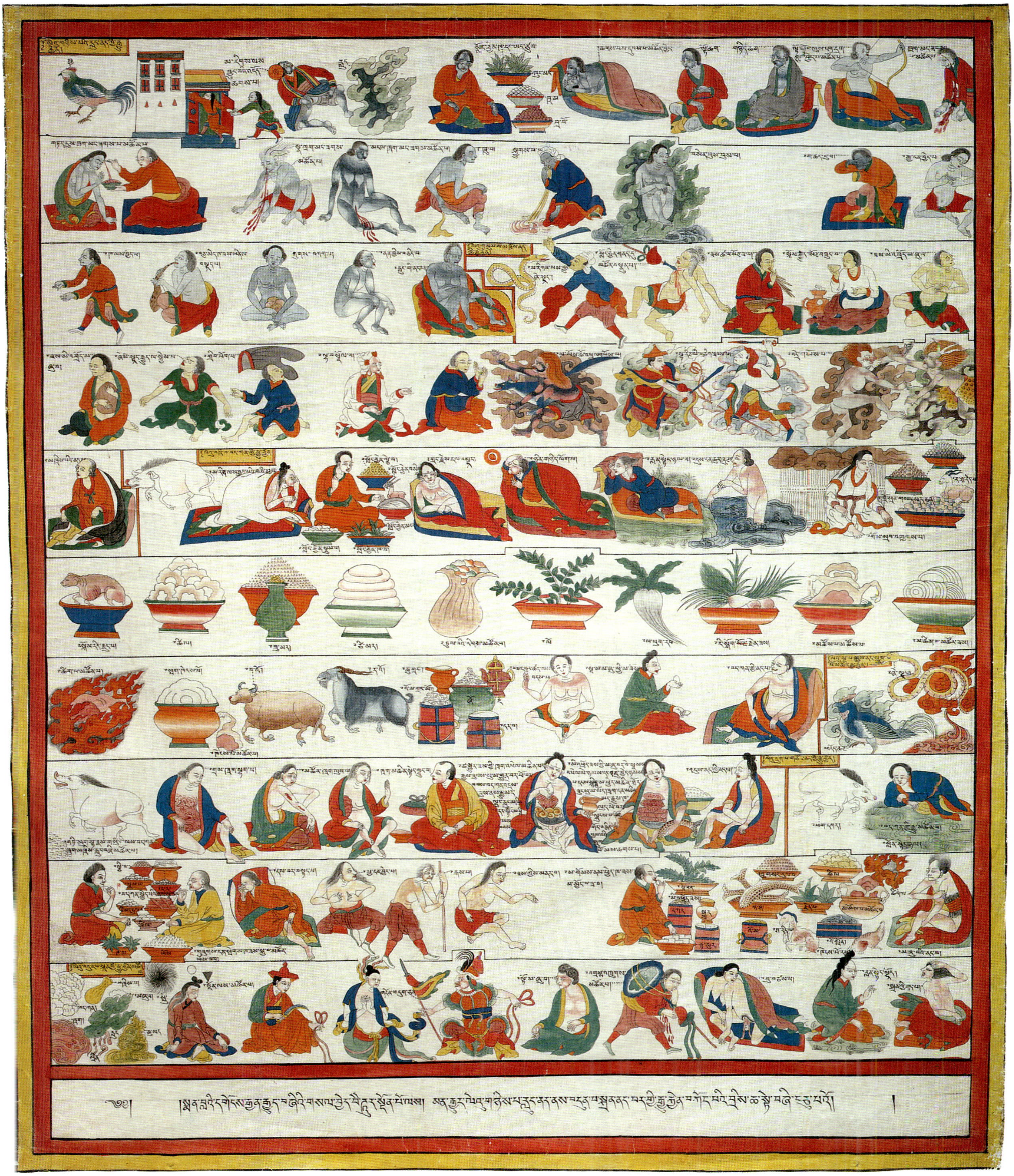

38. Fevers

Diseases that have spread throughout the body must be collected and treated, diseases that are hidden must be brought out and treated, and diseases that have accumulated must be dissolved. This painting illustrates the causes of various types of fevers.

Fever is caused by *mkhris-pa* disorders—for example, by having too much hot potency food and drink such as alcohol, meat, or milk products. It is also caused by too much physical exertion in the midday, autumn, or in a hot climate. This sort of diet and behavior burns the body and imbalances the body temperature. It is like setting a log on a fire.

In Tibetan medicine fever is categorized into nine types:

1. *unripened fever;*
2. *fully developed fever;*
3. *void fever;*
4. *hidden fever;*
5. *chronic fever;*
6. *turbid fever;*
7. *agitated fever;*
8. *traumatic fever; and*
9. *viral fever.*

Unripened fever: Symptoms are a thin, fluttering, and fast pulse. The urine is red-yellow, turbid, and thick; there are small red rashes on the tongue; the body temperature fluctuates; there is a bitter taste in the mouth, tiredness, chills, and confusing dreams at night.

Fully developed fever: Symptoms are a pulse that is bulky, strong, rolling, firm, and fast. The urine is red-yellow and there is a strong odor and vapor; there is heaviness in the body, a loss of appetite, thirst, sweating, headaches, and delirium.

Void fever: The pulse is empty and flowing. The patient experiences breathlessness, has red eyes, and the tongue is red, dry, and coarse. There is shifting pain throughout the body, thirst, snoring, and loss of sleep.

Hidden fever: The pulse is shallow and taut, the urine is red, the face is oily, after getting out of bed in the morning the mouth and tongue are dry, with a bitter taste. There is a loss of appetite, heavy head, nose bleeding, heavy sleep in the daytime, and light sleep at night.

Chronic fever: The pulse is thin and fast, the urine is red and its vapor disappears slowly. The lips stick together; the palate is dry and stiff; and the eyes are red, dry, and watery. There is a blueish complexion, and palpitation and breathlessness after only a little physical movement. There is numbness in the limbs and heaviness in the lower body, and there is a continual craving for cold water.

Turbid fever: The pulse is thin, fast, and deeply flowing. The urine is red and the face looks swollen and pale; the tongue, gums, and nails lose their color. There is profuse sweating, a dry tongue and mouth, constant coughing, and heavy sleep. The legs and eyes are swollen, and the body becomes overly sensitive. Turbid fever is caused by an imbalance of serum and if left untreated it can lead to the formation of pus in the full organs, such as in the lungs.

Agitated fever: The pulse is bulky, strong, firm, and fast. The urine is red-yellow and the odor and vapor are strong. The patient has chills and short sharp pains, difficulty moving, and red-yellow and blackish sputum.

Traumatic fever is caused by trauma in the five full and six hollow organs. The pulse is fast and thin, the urine is red and has a strong odor. The traumatized organ is painful and sensitive. For example, if the heart is traumatized, speech is affected and it becomes difficult for the patient to focus. There is constant pain in the heart. The patient will stare, unblinking, and sometimes faint.

Viral fever: The patient experiences similar symptoms as those described for unripened, developed, and void fevers. There will also be constant pain in the back, hips, and joints; loss of appetite; headaches; chills; and a lack of sleep.

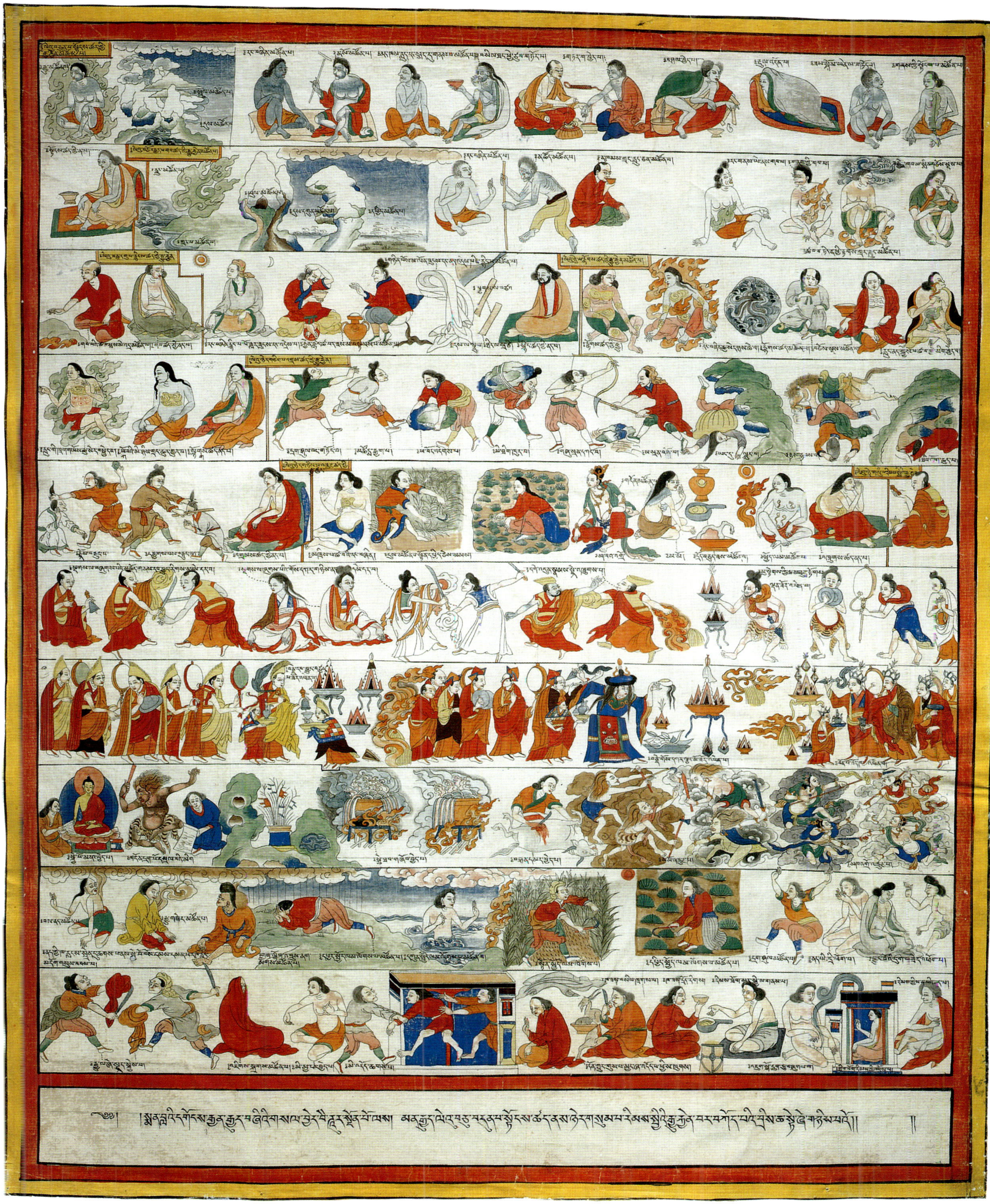

39. Gynecological and Obstetric Diseases; Madness; Epilepsy, Stroke; Plagues

This painting shows various gynecological diseases connected with the female body. Because women have breasts and wombs and undergo a menstrual cycle, there are various diseases connected with these.

Uterine diseases are associated with *rlung, mkhris-pa, bad-kan,* blood, and a combination of all four. There are ten diseases connected with amenorrhea or menorrhagia *(khrag-tshabs)* related to the lungs, heart, liver, spleen, gall bladder, kidneys, small intestine, breasts, and menstrual cycle.

Specific gynecological diseases include the chronic *khrag-tshabs* called *rlung-tshabs,* related to symptoms of the head, bones, heart, kidney, stomach, and small intestines. There are also nine uterine tumors and two diseases connected with disturbance of microorganisms.

There are common gynecological and obstetric diseases related to pregnancy, abortion, breech birth, extracting placenta, uterine prolapse, postnatal hemorrhage, postnatal disease, and postnatal infection. The last is caused by eating too much heat-producing food such as meat, alcohol, and butter, and by sleeping in the daytime—these increase body heat and imbalance *mkhris-pa.*

Diseases caused by demons include possession by evil spirits, madness, dementia, epilepsy, and leprosy.

For example, the causes of madness are shown in the fifth and sixth rows: low self-esteem, grief, unhappiness, mental stress, incompatible diet, and poor behavior. These all contribute to the disturbance of the three *nyes-pas,* and disrupt the channels of consciousness. They dim the memory, and the person's mind loses its ability to function normally. There are seven types of madness: *rlung* madness, *mkhris-pa* madness, *bad-kan* madness, a combination of those three, mental distress, madness caused by poisons, and demonic possession. When the madness is of the *rlung* type, the patient has the following symptoms: weight loss, emitting foamy vomit, excessive talking and crying, the scleras of the eyes are red, and they suffer postdigestive pain. *Mkhris-pa* madness is identified by a very short temper, violence, a craving for cold food and drink, and seeing fires and stars. *Bad-kan* madness is reserved: the patient sleeps heavily, has no appetite, excess saliva, and a runny nose. The madness that is a combination of *rlung, mkhris-pa,* and *bad-kan* is indicated by all the above symptoms.

People suffering from mental distress get worse when they think of lost lovers or lost business; when thinking about these and other regrets, they cry and faint. For people suffering from madness caused by poisons, the poisons affect the whole bodily system; their complexion is drained of all life; and they become delirious and hallucinate, leading to dullness of the mind. People suffering from demonic possession completely change their behavior.

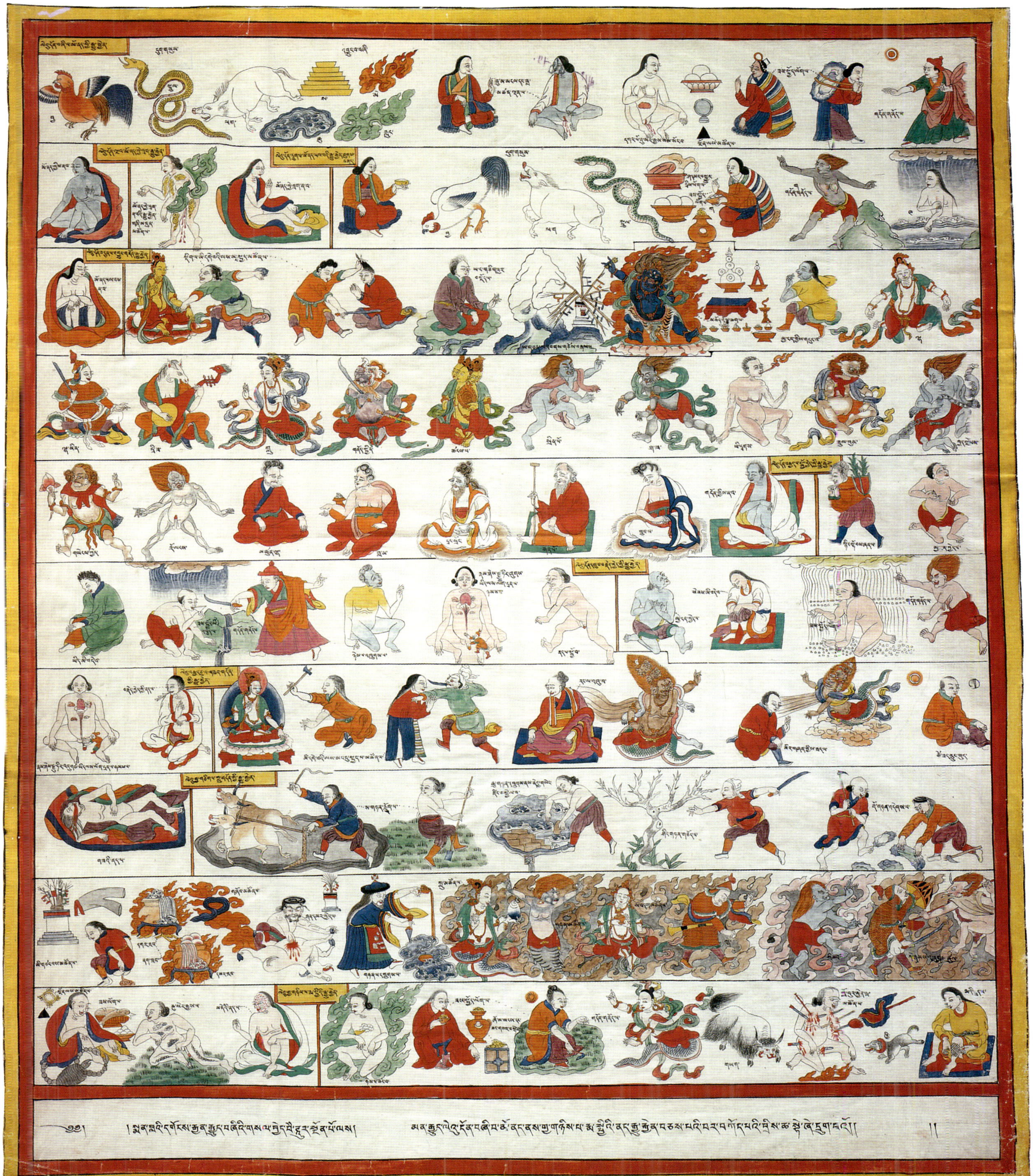

40. The Physician

To heal the disease of the patient the most important person is the physician. This painting deals with the qualities required in a physician, the level of knowledge of the physician, the definition of a physician, different types of physicians, what the physician actually does, and the rewards of being a good physician.

A physician will have an analytical mind that has learned the *Four Tantras* and has developed some intuitive knowledge. The physician will be compassionate, possessing a good heart and treating all patients equally, as if treating his own mother. He will respect medical ethics and be committed to his profession. Also important are respect for gurus, teachers, medical instruments, and fellow physicians; to have no revulsion when seeing the pus, blood, urine, feces, and vomit of patients; to consider all the medicines and medical scriptures as wish-fulfilling jewels; and to ensure that all medicines are blessed according to proper Buddhist ritual. The physician must be very patient in body, speech, and mind. Patience through the body is expressed by making medicine carefully; patience through speech by making the patient happy, relaxed, and comfortable; and patience through the mind by being alert and able to accurately diagnose and treat the disease of the patient. Continuous effort is required to learn and gain more experience. The concentration required when seeing a patient is the same as the concentration needed by a person who is walking on a wall, with a bowl of melted butter on his head, threatened with death if a single drop is spilled. The physician should be both gentle and contented, and helpful toward the destitute. The physician should know by heart the causative factors of diseases and their proper treatment.

The definition of a physician is one who heals all pain and practices medicine to promote good health. When performing surgery the doctor should be as confident and courageous as a father saving his child. In the reign of King Songtsen Gampo in seventh-century Tibet, doctors were known as *Lha-je,* the king's king.

Different types of physicians are divided into topmost, special, and ordinary. The topmost *(mempa lha-na-mehpa)* are like the Healing Buddha, possessing omniscient knowledge. The special *(mempa khepar)* possess intuitive knowledge and they able to generate strong compassion to help the suffering of the patient.

The bottom half of the painting metaphorically illustrates the necessary qualities of a good physician. The ordinary physician *(mempa phelpa)* must have an authentic link with a teacher—otherwise he resembles a fox seizing a king's throne; without a link with a teacher the physician will garner no respect. The physician must have studied the *Four Tantras*—otherwise it is like showing objects to someone who is blind; the physician will not know how to treat and diagnose. A physician with no skills or experience is like someone on an unknown path; the physician will have no confidence and will be full of doubt. A physician who is unable to diagnose illness is like someone wandering in a foreign country without friends; he will be unable to distinguish a single disease. A physician who is unable to read the pulse or perform uroscopy is like a spy unable to send a secret message; the physician will not know whether the patient has a cold disease or hot disease. A physician who is unable to comment on or predict the outcome of disease is like a chieftan who cannot give a speech to his clan; the physician will gain a bad reputation. A physician who does not know how to treat the patient resembles someone who shoots at a target in the dark; the physician is unable to get any

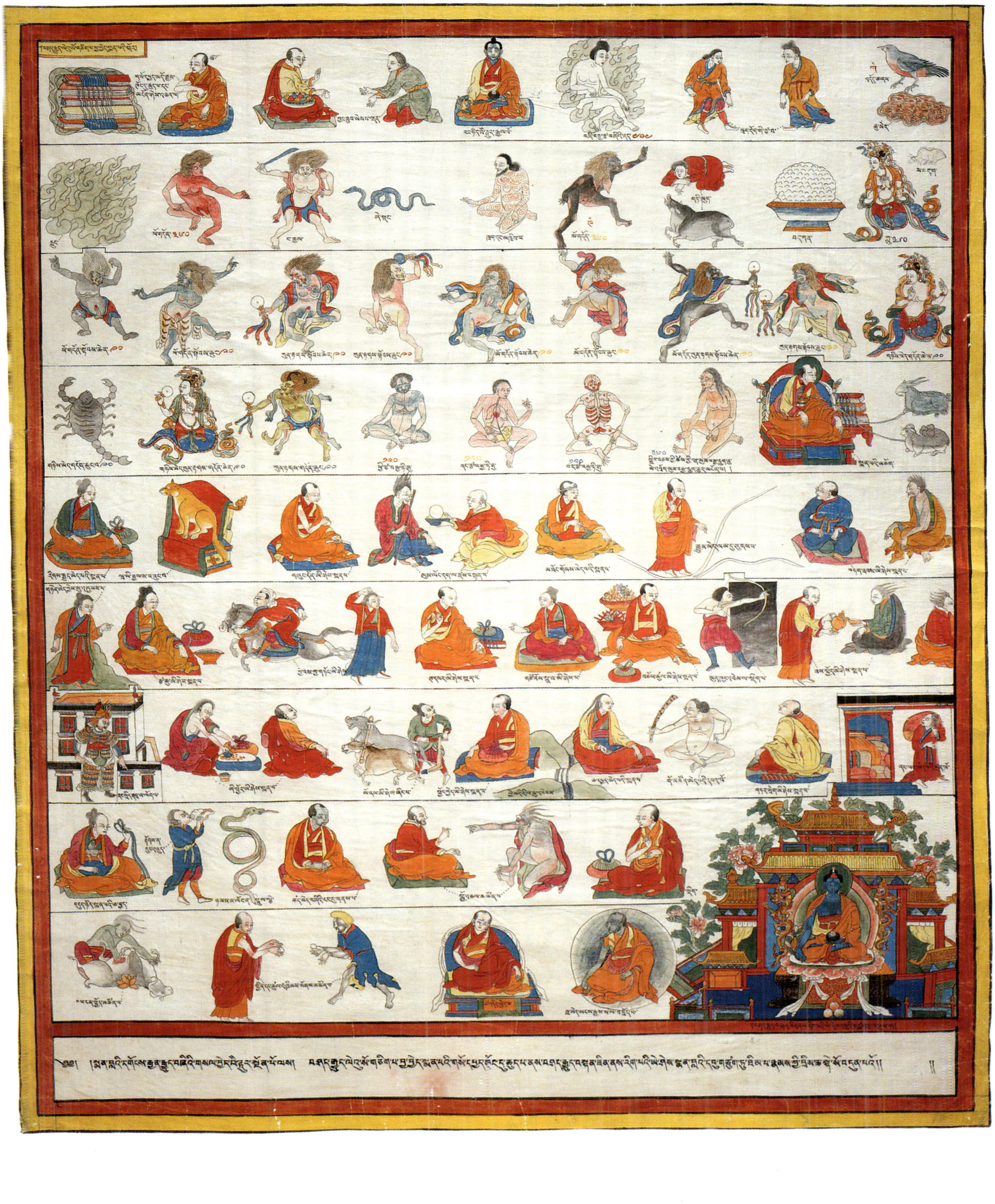

response from his efforts. A physician with no knowledge of diet and conduct is like a king who is opposed by his subjects; the patient eats the wrong food and does the wrong things, and wrecks the bodily constitution. A physician who cannot prepare medicine is like a farmer who does not how to cultivate the land; wrongly prepared medicine can disturb the whole system and cause various side effects. A physician who cannot prepare cathartic medicinal compounds is like someone pouring water onto a mound of sand where nothing will come out; if emetics are being used they will not work. A physician with no medical instruments or medicine is like a courageous warrior going to war with no weapons; the physician is unable to eliminate any diseases. Finally, the physician wo has no knowledge of bloodletting and moxibustion is like a thief who has no knowledge of where the valuables are stored; the physician cannot use the moxibustion and bloodletting points of the body. It is important to avoid such physicians—they are said to be like demons of death in the guise of doctors.

Physicians should try to collect as much medicine as possible in order to prescribe the right kind of medicine for disease. They must always think about the needs of the patient, and they should always be available. They should be able to predict whether the disease of the patient is curable or not. They should possess the six perfections of generosity, ethics, patience, effort, concentration, and wisdom.

The short-term results of being an excellent physician are happiness, wealth, and a good reputation. In the long term, if the physician is fully motivated and concentrated on healing patients, he will achieve enlightenment in this life simply by treating patients.

Glossary

Abhidharmakosha: The *Abhidharmakosha,* a philosophical treatise written by Vasubandhu (probably Vasubandhu the Younger, who is said to have lived in the fifth century C.E.), expounds the idea that everything in the past, present, and future exists at once. The treatise is a compilation of the teachings of the Sarvastivada school of Buddhism, which was a transition between the Hinayana ("small vehicle") and Mahayana ("great vehicle") views, and commentaries on the teachings.

Amitabha: In Mahayana Buddhism, Amitabha is one of the five Buddhas traditionally pictured in mandalas representing the divisions of the Buddha-nature. Amitabha is the king of the pure western paradise called Sukhavati, "The Land of Bliss."

Astangahrdaya Samhita: One of the medical texts included in the *Tangyur* attributed to Vagbhata, a seventh-century Indian doctor. It is also one of the basic sources used in the compilation of the *Four Tantras.*

atman: In Hinduism, *atman* signifies the essential self—similar to the Western notion of the soul—that is pure, subtle, and eternal. Buddhism does not recognize the existence of *atman,* or the self. This doctrine of nonself, one of the central ideas in Buddhism, is called *anatman:* there is no existing, permanent, independent part of a being; rather the essential nature of a being is changeable and prone to suffering.

avatara: From Sanskrit root meaning "to descend," the incarnation of a god or deity.

Ayurveda: The traditional system of medicine in India, Ayurveda (from Sanskrit "knowledge of longevity" or "knowledge of life") was codified in the first centuries of this era. The main Ayurvedic texts are the *Caraka Samhita* and the *Susruta Samhita,* which detail a physiological system based on the three humors *(dosas)* similar to bile, wind, and phlegm. These long texts include chapters on the characteristics and treatment of diseases, diet, medicinal plants, anatomy, and surgical techniques.

bad-kan: One of the three humors in Tibetan medicine, *bad-kan* (pronounced "baygan") helps sustain bodily fluids and is equivalent to phlegm. It is associated with the properties of earth and water. There are five kinds of *bad-kan*—supporting, decomposing, experiencing, satisfying, and connecting—that aid different aspects of the body and bodily functions.

Bardo thödol: Known in English as the *Tibetan Book of the Dead,* this Buddhist scripture describing the phases of death is attributed to Padmasambhava. The title is literally translated as "Liberation in the Intermediate State Through Hearing."

bardo: Literally "between," an in-between state. There are six kinds of *bardo* as described in the *Naro chödrug* (which details important meditation techniques) and in the *Bardo thödol:* the *bardos* of birth, dreams, meditation, and the three dreamlike stages of *bardo* from the moment of death to rebirth.

Bhaisajyaguru: The Healing Buddha *(see).*

bla: Life energy that flows through the three lifespan channels; the physician can feel the patient's *bla* in the third lifespan channel as it passes through the wrist.

Blue Beryl: The commentary written by Sangye Gyamtso in the seventeenth century to accompany his revised edition of the *Four Tantras (Gyushi).* In the medical paintings presented here, the text at the bottom is usually an excerpt from the *Blue Beryl* that explains the chapters illustrated in each painting.

bodhi: Literally "awakened," Sanskrit term for enlightenment.

bodhisattva: Enlightened being—or Buddha-to-be—who decides to stay in the world to help all sentient beings achieve their own enlightenment and escape suffering. According to Sutra tradition, the path of a bodhisattva takes millions of lifetimes.

bodily constituents: According to Tibetan medicine, there are seven principle substances that constitute the body: nutritional "essence" from ingested food, blood, flesh, fat, bone, and the reproductive fluids (semen and menstrual blood).

Bön: The pre-Buddhist indigenous religious tradition of Tibet. Bön developed a large body of literature and an institutional structure similar to those of Tibetan Buddhism.

Buryatia: Located in the southern area of eastern Siberia between Mongolia and Lake Baikal, Buryatia has been part of the multinational Russian empire since the mid-seventeenth century. In 1923, the Buryat-Mongol Autonomous Soviet Socialist Republic (ASSR) was established as part of the USSR. Since 1992, the Republic of Buryatia has been part of the Russian Federation.

Caraka Samhita: One of the two earliest Sanskrit texts to outline the Ayurvedic system of Indian medicine. The *Caraka Samhita* is unusual in that in addition to medicine, it also deals with the philosophical doctrines of *samkhya* and *vaisesika,* although it was written prior to the standard texts of these doctrines.

cauterization: External therapy used as a last resort to treat wounds or abscesses.

Chagpori: The famed medical college on top of the Iron Hill

on the outskirts of Lhasa, Tibet. It was built in the seventeenth century by the regent Sangye Gyamtso, and destroyed by the Chinese in 1959.

Chakpa Chophel: The main disciple of Sangye Gyamtso.

chakra: Sanskrit term, literally "wheel," for an energy point in the body where different channels intertwine; the *chakras* are visualized in Buddhist meditation. In Tibetan Buddhism there are five *chakras* (sometimes only the first three are used), each of which is centered in a different part of the body and represents an aspect of the Buddha: the *chakras* of Bliss (located in the head, representing the body aspect), Enjoyment (in the throat, representing speech), Phenomena (in the heart, representing mind), Transmutation (in the navel, representing quality), and Preservation of Happiness (in the genitals, representing activity). Each of the *chakras* also has a corresponding meditational syllable: head = OM, throat = AH, heart = HUM, navel = SWA, genitals = HA. For a complete description of the *chakras,* see Clifford, pp. 73–76.

chakravartin: Sanskrit term, literally "wheel ruler," for a world ruler or buddha whose teaching is applicable to the entire universe.

Chandrabhinandana (eighth century): According to one version of the story of the origin of the *Four Tantras,* Chandrabhinandana collaborated in the translation of this text from Sanskrit into Tibetan.

Chang school: One of the two schools of Tibetan medicine after a split in the fourteenth century; the tradition based on the Chang lineage was followed mainly in the north.

channels *(rtsa):* Pathways for different kinds of wind and other substances (illustrated in plate 6), they consist of the embryonic formation channels, existent channels, connecting channels (also illustrated in plates 7 and 8), and lifespan channels (also in plate 7). Where the channels intertwine at various points throughout the body, *chakras* are formed—many yoga exercises are designed to loosen constricted *chakras.* See also *subtle channels.*

Dalai Lama: The spiritual and secular leader of Tibet, thought to be the reincarnation of the bodhisattva Avalokiteshvara. The full title is Dalai Lama Vajradhara (Lama, Ocean [of Wisdom], Holder of the Thunderbolt). *Dalai* means "oceanic" in Mongolian. Lama is the Tibetan term for guru, "spiritual teacher." The title was first given to Sonam Gyatso, a reincarnated lama of the Gelugpa order, by Mongol chief Altan Khan in 1578 as an honorific title. The Fifth Dalai Lama (Losang Gyatso, 1617–82) was the first who was invested with both spiritual and secular authority, in 1642, with the help of the Mongols.

dbang: Tantric initiation conveyed by a Tantric master to a fully prepared disciple, empowering him or her to practice one of the Tantric meditation practices.

decoction: An extract made by boiling and concentrating various substances, such as herbs, to be used as medicine.

dharani: Short sutras containing sets of syllables, similar to mantras, that are repeated in order to attain certain states of mind.

Dharma: The teachings of the Buddha, or the doctrines of Buddhism. In India, Buddhism was known as Buddhadharma.

Dharamsala: In Himachal Pradesh, India, the city of Dharamsala is the seat of the Tibetan government in exile and the temporary home of His Holiness the Dalai Lama.

dhatu: Sanskrit term, literally "element, realm." It is the sensory aspect of the eighteenth-century Tibetan classification of sciences called *The Eighteeen Spheres of Knowledge of the Inner and Outer World of Man.*

Dri-med: The commentary on the *Kalachakra Tantra.*

emchi: Tibetan term for doctor.

evacuation remedies: Extensively used treatments including purgatives, emetics, medicinal snuffs, and mild and strong enemas.

Explanatory Tantra: One of the volumes of the *Four Tantras,* the Explanatory Tantra completely outlines the Tibetan medical doctrine, including subjects such as embryology, anatomy, pathology, conduct and diet, *materia medica* and medical instruments, diagnosis and treatment of specific disorders, and medical ethics. In the first chapter (illustrated in plate 3), an emanation of the Buddha, Vidyajnana, flows out of the crown of the Healing Buddha to present the tantra. At the conclusion of the Explanatory Tantra (illustrated in plate 40), Vidyajnana is absorbed back into the crown of the Healing Buddha.

fomentation: Fomentation treatment can consist of soaking in a bath (preferably a natural hot springs, but a hot bath spiked with the appropriate medicinal plants and substances will do), or applying hot, moist packs directly on the body. Fomentation is used to treat fevers, old wounds, ulcers, channel disorders, swelling, atrophy and stiffness of the muscles, and so on.

four medical traditions: When the Buddha Shakyamuni was said to have taught the medical tantras, the disciples heard the teachings differently according to their varying modes of understanding. The gods heard the teachings as "The Jug of Cure," the sages heard it as "The Eight Works of Charaka," the non-Buddhists heard it as "The Tantra of the Black Shiva," and the Buddhists heard it as "The Teachings of the Three Protectors."

Four Tantras (Gyushi): The fundamental text of Tibetan medicine. Its origins are obscure, but Buddhist tradition attributes it to Shakyamuni, who manifested as the Healing Buddha in India and whose teachings were recorded in Sanskrit. The historical theory is that it was written by a Tibetan, possibly Yuthog the Younger, in the twelfth century—and not translated from Sanskrit. It is composed of four volumes: the Root Tantra, Explanatory Tantra, Instructional Tantra, and the Subsequent Tantra.

full organs (also called solid or vital organs): heart, lungs, liver, spleen, and kidneys.

Galen (c. 130–c. 200 C.E.): Greek physician in the court of the Roman emperor who refined the humoral theory developed by the Hippocratic school.

Gelugpa: School of Tibetan Buddhism founded by Tsong Khapa (1357–1419), also known as the yellow-hat sect. The Gelugpa school was the latest to develop in Tibet, and since the seventeenth century the Gelugpas have held the most important political positions. The doctrine emphasizes intense study of Buddhist texts and monastic rigor.

Genyen of Lhasa: According to the colophon of the *Atlas of Tibetan Medicine,* Gen'en was the colorist for the original set of paintings.

Gyushi: the *Four Tantras (see).*

Healing Buddha: Bhaisajyaguru, said to be the manifestation that the Buddha assumed when he taught the medical tantras. Also known as Vaiduryaprabha. Aspects of the ultimate Buddha-nature are also manifested in Buddhas such as Mañjushri (wisdom), Vajrapani (power), and Avalokiteshvara (compassion).

Hippocrates (c. 460–c. 377 B.C.E.): Greek physician generally known as the founder of Western medicine.

hollow organs: stomach, small intestine, large intestine, gall bladder, urinary bladder, and reproductive organs.

humors *(nyes-pas):* The elements that are involved in the physiological processes of the body. In Tibetan medicine they are *rlung* (wind/movement), *mkhris-pa* (bile/heat), and *bad-kan* (phlegm/water/earth). When they are in equilibrium, the person is healthy; disease is a result of the aggravation or imbalance of the three humors.

Kalachakra Tantra: Literally "tantra of the wheel of time," an important tenth-century tantra dealing with cosmology and an apocalyptic view of time, considered to be the basis of the Tibetan calendar. Its transmission is connected with the mythical kingdom of Shambhala.

Kangyur: The Tibetan Buddhist canon that contains the words of the Buddha Shakyamuni. Translated from Sanskrit, it is comprised of 108 volumes. (See *Tangyur.*)

karma: A central theory of Buddhism; the law of cause and effect. Virtuous actions result in happiness in this life or in a future life, and nonvirtuous actions result in suffering. In Tibetan medicine, some diseases are considered to be karmic, the inevitable result of some past action in the present life or in a past life; the patient will not respond to medical treatment. In the case of karmic diseases, the only remedy is the practice of Dharma, the Buddha's teaching.

Khanbo Lama: Buryat-Mongolian title for a high-ranking lama.

Khogbug: Sangye Gyamtso's treatise on the history of medicine, written around the end of the seventeenth century.

King Trisong Detsen (742–97): King of Tibet and the restorer of Buddhism in Tibet. Like the earlier King Songtsen Gampo, he summoned physicians from surrounding regions.

lama: Tibetan term for guru (Sanskrit), a spiritual teacher or mentor.

Lhantab: A supplement to the third volume of the *Four Tantras,* added by Sangye Gyamtso.

lokayata: A school of Hinduism whose teaching emphasizes materialism.

Manasija: The Born Sage of the Spirit, said to be the only disciple to have understood the whole teaching as the *Four Tantras* when Shakyamuni delivered it. He is depicted second from the left in the upper register of the second painting (plate 2), requesting the teaching from the Healing Buddha. He is said to be an emanation of the Healing Buddha's speech.

mandala: A Buddha's palace, literally "circle." Mandalas can be depicted in three- or two-dimensional form, the latter rendered in paint or sand. The mandala features its main buddha on a throne in the center, surrounded by other buddhas, bodhisattvas, and deities.

mantra: A set of syllables recited in Buddhist meditation. For example, the mantra OM MANE PADME HUM is used to call upon the bodhisattva of compassion.

Mendzekhang: The School of Medicine and Astrology in Lhasa, Tibet. The medical college was founded in 1916 by the Thirteenth Dalai Lama.

mkhris-pa: One of the three humors in Tibetan medicine, *mkhris-pa* (pronounced "treeba") is the heat that regulates body temperature and aids digestion, equivalent to bile. It is associated with the properties of fire. There are five kinds of *mkhris-pa*—digestive, determining, complexion-clearing, sight-enhancing, and color-regulating—that are responsible for different aspects of the body and bodily functions.

moxibustion: The therapeutic technique of moxibustion was introduced to Tibetan medicine from China. Cylinders of dried gerbera leaves or a mixture of several herbs are affixed to or held over the specific moxibustion points on the body, then ignited. Sometimes the moxa cone is attached with a needle—similar to an acupuncture needle—and the heat from the burning cone is conducted into the flesh. It is considered to be effective for treating cold and damp diseases such as rheumatism.

myrobalan: Considered a remedy for almost all diseases, the fruit, stem, roots, and flowers of the myrobalan tree *(Terminalia chebula)* are used extensively in Tibetan medicine. The Healing Buddha is often depicted holding a branch of myrobalan.

nagas: In Tibetan Buddhism, *nagas* are water deities who guard certain teachings of the Buddha in underwater palaces until humanity is ready to receive them.

nirvana: Literally "extinction," the final release from the

endless cycle of death and rebirth through the extinction of all passions, illusions, and desires; a oneness with the absolute; a place of salvation; bliss.

nyes-pas: Humors *(see).*

Oddiyana: An area in Swat, Pakistan, believed to be the birthplace of Padmasambhava and the Buddhist tantra. Some people believe it is the location of the Palace of Bhaisajyaguru, the Healing Buddha.

Padmasambhava: An Indian Great Adept of Buddhism, known to Tibetans as the Second Buddha. He was invited to Tibet by the king in 749 to help establish Samye *(bsam-yas),* the first Buddhist monastery in Tibet. He is credited with the authorship of many texts, including the *Bardo thödol,* known in English as the *Tibetan Book of the Dead.*

Panchen Lama: Literally "great scholar," the second-highest spiritual dignitary in Tibetan Buddhism, revered as the incarnation of the Buddha Amitabha. The panchen lamas' monastery traditionally has been the Tashi Lhunpo Monastery. The theory of the Panchen incarnations was started by the Fifth Dalai Lama and continues to this day.

Potala Palace: Official winter residence of the Dalai Lama in Lhasa, Tibet, built by the Fifth Dalai Lama beginning in about 1645.

potencies: The eight potencies recognized in Tibetan pharmacology are affected by the tastes, and therefore by the elements. They are expressed as opposites: heavy/light, unctuous/rough, cold/hot, and dull/sharp.

prana: Literally "breath of life," in Hinduism the life force or energy that permeates the body, physically manifest as the breath.

preta: Literally "departed one." Rebirth as a *preta,* sometimes thought of as a hungry ghost because he must suffer tortures such as hunger, is the result of karma that is not good enough for rebirth into one of the more positive modes of existence.

Qing Dynasty: Chinese dynasty that lasted from 1644 to 1912.

rishi: Originally a sage or a seer to whom the hymns of the Vedas were revealed, today the term is applied to poets, philosophers, and sages.

rlung: One of the three humors in Tibetan medicine, *rlung* (pronounced "loong") is associated with the properties of air and represents the wind *nyes-pa* in the body. There are various types of *rlung*—ascending, downward-cleansing, pervasive, and fire-accompanying—that aid different bodily functions.

Root Tantra: The first volume of the *Four Tantras,* the Root Tantra outlines the entire Tibetan medical system, including a general introduction, physiology and pathology, diagnosis, and treatment (plates 1, 2, 13, and 19). In the paintings presented here, the medical system is illustrated as a series of trees.

rtsa: Channels *(see).*

Sakyapa: One of the four major sects of Tibetan Buddhism, named after the Sakya ("grey earth") monastery in western Tibet.

samsara: The cycle of perpetual transmigration in which the soul of a living being dies and is reborn; the wheel of existence.

Sangye Gyamtso (1653–1705): Regent of the Fifth Dalai Lama, physician, and medical historian, he wrote the *Blue Beryl* treatise, the commentary on the *Four Tantras.* He organized the revision of the *Four Tantras,* and was involved in commissioning the illustrations, later copies of which are presented in this volume. He also founded the Chagpori medical college in Lhasa.

Shakyamuni Buddha: The epithet of Siddhartha Gautama (566 or 563–486 or 483 B.C.E.), the founder of Buddhism, the historical Buddha. Siddhartha, a prince of the Shakya clan in the city of Kapilavastu in what is now Nepal, failed to achieve enlightenment through the practice of esceticism, so he left his teachers and turned to meditation. He achieved complete *bodhi* when he was thirty-five and eventually began to teach to a growing number of disciples, who gave him the title Shakyamuni Buddha. His life story is now infused with mythic and spiritual elements, and some of the most beautiful Buddhist literature is devoted to meditational descriptions of offerings made to the Buddha at his celestial palace.

Songtsen Gampo: King of Tibet in the early seventh century. During his reign a form of Tibetan script was developed, and he commissioned physicians from India, China, and Iran to write texts concerning their different medical traditions.

soothing remedies: decoctions, medicinal powders, pills, pastes, sugars or fats, medicinal beverages, gemstone medications, and herbal compounds.

sowa rigpa: Tibetan for "the science of healing."

Subsequent Tantra: The last volume of the *Four Tantras,* it explains the practical application of pulse examination, uroscopy, tongue examination, oil therapy, cathartic procedures, bloodletting, moxibustion, and other treatments. Also called the *Last Tantra.*

subtle channels: The three main subtle channels—*Roma, rKyang-ma,* and *dBu-ma*—are not fully described in the medical tantras. In Tibetan medicine they do not necessarily correspond to the physical veins in the body; rather, they are more like psychic channels. *Roma* is influenced by the sun, *rKyang-ma* by the moon, and *dBu-ma* by neutral energy.

Sudarsana: Mythical city of medicine (literally "beautiful to behold") where the Healing Buddha is said to have taught (see plate 1).

Susruta Samhita: One of the two earliest Sanskrit texts to outline the Ayurvedic system of Indian medicine. The *Susruta Samhita* is of special interest to medical historians because it contains specific instructions for complicated and relatively advanced surgical procedures.

sutra: Sanskrit term, literally "aphorism." A teaching considered to be taught by the Buddha himself or with his sanction.

Taittiriya-Upanishad: One of the earliest Upanishads, it discusses the five elements that compose a living being: matter *(prakriti)*, life *(prana)*, consciousness *(manas)*, intelligence *(vijnana)*, and bliss *(ananda)*.

Tangyur: Commentaries on the *Kangyur*. It contains not only the Buddhist exegesis but also treatises on the sciences.

tantra: The use of elaborate rituals in Buddhism and Hinduism adapted from ancient religious practices and techniques in India using magical and sexual symbolism. The term also refers to specific texts describing the path, techniques (such as yoga), and practice of a particular teaching, using mantras and mandala depictions.

Tara: A female bodhisattva of compassion who was widely worshipped—and her mantra widely recited—in Tibet. Also known as Drolma, the Mother of Buddhas, Tara represents the feminine aspect of the Buddha, and the wisdom of emptiness.

tastes: The six tastes recognized in Tibetan pharmacology result from combinations of two of the elements of earth, water, fire, and wind. Excess intake of foods with these tastes significantly affects the humors: a sweet taste reduces *rlung* and *mkhris-pa,* acidic reduces *rlung* and *bad-kan,* salty reduces *rlung* and *bad-kan,* bitter reduces *mkhris-pa,* hot reduces *rlung* and *bad-kan,* and astringent reduces *mkhris-pa.*

Tendzin Norbuchen of Lhobrag: Said to be the draftsman of the *Atlas of Tibetan Medicine.*

thangka: Tibetan iconic painting.

Three Jewels: The Buddha, his Dharma, and the Sangha (followers of Buddhism, including monks, nuns, and laity). A Buddhist seeks refuge in the Three Jewels rather than in worldly goods.

Three Protectors: Mañjushri (embodying wisdom), Avalokiteshvara (embodying compassion), and Vajrapani (embodying power).

three poisons: According to Buddhist philosophy and medicine, the three negative mindsets of delusion or ignorance *(gTi-mug)*, desire or lust *('Dod-chags)*, and hatred or anger *(Zhe-sdang)* motivate all nonvirtuous actions and are the cause of all suffering (see the three leaves in the center of plate 2). During the formation of the fetus, the three poisons become associated with—and contaminate—the three humors of *bad-kan, rlung,* and *mkhris-pa,* respectively, thus linking Buddhist philosophy with the humoral system. In Buddhist iconography, delusion in represented as a pig, desire as a cock, and hatred as a snake (see plate 37, on the far right of the seventh row and the far left of the eighth row).

Upanishads: Ancient Indian philosophical texts dealing with metaphysical speculations, composed during the first millennium B.C.E.

Vaidurya ngonpo: The Tibetan title of the *Blue Beryl* treatise *(see)*.

Vairocana: According to one story of the origin of the *Four Tantras,* Vairocana translated them from Sanskrit into Tibetan and carried the text to Tibet from India in the eighth century. Another version of the story claims that the *Four Tantras* were actually first written in Tibetan by Yuthog Yontan Gonpo the Younger.

vaisheshika: The oldest school of Hindu philosophy, primarily scientific in its focus.

Vedas: The earliest sacred Indian scriptures; the four Vedas were first transmitted orally, then written in Sanskrit. The Vedic era in India is considered to be from 1500 to 500 B.C.E.

vyakarana: The study of grammar (Sanskrit). *Vyakarana* is covered in one part of the Hindu Vedangas, supplementary texts to the Vedas.

White Beryl: Treatise on astrology written in 1685 by Sangye Gyamtso.

Yellow Beryl: Treatise on the history of Tibet written in 1698 by Sangye Gyamtso.

yoga: Sanskrit term meaning "a yoking," any mental or physical act of discipline by which one becomes yoked, or bound, to the divine as a means of salvation.

Yuan Dynasty: The Mongol dynasty that lasted from 1260 to 1368, founded by Kublai Khan.

Yuthog Yontan Gonpo the Younger (twelfth century): He and his ancestor, who is said to have lived in the eighth century, were accomplished tantric masters, according to Tibetan mythic tradition. Yuthog the Younger was the possible author of the *Four Tantras.* He is regarded as a reincarnation of the Healing Buddha.

Zur: One of the two schools of Tibetan medicine after a split in the fourteenth century, the tradition based on the Zur lineage was followed mainly in the south.

List of Works Illustrated

Note: Plate numbers precede the titles; the numbers in brackets refer to the numbering system used in Tibetan Medical Paintings *(Harry N. Abrams, 1992).*

Selected Bibliography

Tibetan Medicine

Aris, Anthony and Jan Van Alphen, eds. *Oriental Medicine: An Illustrated Guide to the Asian Arts of Healing.* London: Serindia Publications, 1995.

Aschoff, Jürgen C. *Annotated Bibliography of Tibetan Medicine.* Ulm, Germany: Fabri Verlag, 1996.

———. *Tibetan Medicine: East Meets West—West Meets East.* Ulm, Germany: Fabri Verlag, 1993.

Birnbaum, Raoul. *The Healing Buddha.* Boulder, Colorado: Shambhala Publications, Inc., 1979.

Clark, Barry, trans. *The Quintessence Tantras of Tibetan Medicine.* Ithaca, New York: Snow Lion Publications, 1995.

Clifford, Terry. *Tibetan Buddhist Medicine and Psychiatry: The Diamond Healing.* York Beach, Maine: Samuel Weiser, Inc., second edition 1992.

Dash, VaidyaBhagwan and Doboon Tulku. *Positive Health in Tibetan Medicine.* Delhi: Sri Satguru Publications, 1991.

Donden, Yeshi. *Health Through Balance: An Introduction to Tibetan Medicine.* Ithaca, New York: Snow Lion Publications, 1986.

Finckh, Elizabeth. *Foundations of Tibetan Medicine,* vol. 1. Translated by Fredericka M. Houser. London: Watkins, 1978.

———. *Studies in Tibetan Medicine.* Ithaca, New York: Snow Lion Publications, 1988.

Goleman, Daniel and Robert A. F. Thurman, eds. *Mind Science: An East-West Dialogue.* Boston: Wisdom Publications, 1991.

Goleman, Daniel, ed. *Healing Emotions: Conversations with the Dalai Lama on Mindfulness, Emotions and Health.* Boston: Shambhala Publications, Inc., 1997.

Mind and Mental Health in Tibetan Medicine. New York: Potala Publications, 1988.

Parfionovitch, Yuri, Fernand Meyer, and Gyurme Dorje, eds. *Tibetan Medical Paintings: Illustrations to the Blue Beryl Treatise of Sangye Gyamtso (1653–1705).* New York: Harry N. Abrams, Inc., 1992.

Reichle, Franz, ed. *The Knowledge of Healing.* Ithaca, New York: Snow Lion Publications, 1997.

Sachs, Robert. *Health for Life: Secrets of Tibetan Ayurveda.* Santa Fe: Clear Light Publishers, 1995.

Thondup, Tulku. *The Healing Power of the Mind: Simple Meditation Exercises for Health, Well-Being, and Enlightenment.* Boston: Shambhala Publications, Inc., 1996.

Tsarong, T. J., trans. and ed. *Fundamentals of Tibetan Medicine.* Dharamsala, India: Tibetan Medical Center, second edition 1995.

Tsarong, T. J., ed. *Handbook of Traditional Tibetan Drugs: Their Nomenclature, Compound, Use, and Dosage.* Kalimpang, India: Tibetan Medical Publications, 1986.

Varela, Francisco, ed. *Sleeping, Dreaming and Dying: An Exploration of Consciousness with the Dalai Lama.* Boston: Wisdom Publications, 1997.

Tibet, Russia, and Buddhism

Avedon, John. *In Exile from the Land of Snows.* New York: Alfred A. Knopf, 1979

Dalai Lama, the Fourteenth. *A Flash of Lightning in the Dark of Night: A Guide to the Bodhisattva Way of Life.* Boston: Shambhala Publications, Inc., 1994.

———. *My Land and My People.* Valois, New York: Gabrial/ Snow Lion Publications, 1962.

Lopez, Donald S., Jr., ed. *Religions of Tibet in Practice.* New Jersey: Princeton University Press, 1997.

Rahula, Walpola. *What the Buddha Taught.* New York: Grove Press, 1974.

Snellgrove, David and Hugh Richardson. *A Cultural History of Tibet.* Boston: Shambhala Publications, Inc., 1980.

Snelling, John. *Buddhism in Russia: The Story of Agvan Dorzhiev, Lhasa's Emissary to the Tsar.* Rockport, Massachusetts: Element, 1993.

Sogyal Rimpoche. *The Tibetan Book of Living and Dying.* San Francisco: HarperSanFrancisco, 1992.

Index

Credits

Photographs of the paintings in the History Museum of Buryatia by Slava Urozaev

Map by Steven Jablonski

Documentary Photographs

Archives, History Museum of Buryatia: pp. 34, 37, 38 (bottom left and right), 40
© Dan Plumley, Consultant on Baikal Programs for Ecologically Sustainable Development: p. 38 (top)
© Franz Reichle, ïThe Knowledge of Healing,î T&C Film AG, Zurich: p. 69 (right)
Tibet Images: pp. 31 (©Kim Yeshi), 36 (© Ernesto Noreiga), 69 (left) (© Markus Bollen), 71 (© Ernesto Noriega)
Col. J. L. R. Weir, CEI. © J. M. Jehu: pp 30, 37 (bottom left)
© Robert Wilkinson, Alternative Energy Specialist for Ecologically Sustainable Development: p. 35

Contributors

John F. Avedon was born in New York and educated at Sarah Lawrence College. He has written for the overseas edition of *Newsweek,* and is the editor of *The Library of Tibet,* a translation series of classic Tibetan texts. His articles on Tibet have appeared in *Geo, Rolling Stone, The New York Times Magazine, Parade,* and *Maclean's.* He presently lives in New York City, and is writing a spiritual biography of the Dalai Lama.

Dr. Natalia D. Bolsokhoeva was born in Ulan-Ude. She graduated from Leningrad University with a specialization in Tibetan medieval literature, and went on to earn a Ph.D. from the Oriental Studies Department of the Russian Academy of Sciences in Moscow. Since 1982, Dr. Bolsokhoeva has been engaged in a scientific study of Tibetan culture, specifically Tibetan medicine, in Nepal. She is the author of three books on Tibetan medicine, one book on Tibetan songs, and more than seventy articles on Tibetan culture. She works at the Institute of Social Sciences of the Siberian Branch of the Russian Academy of Sciences.

Dr. Tamdin Sither Bradley was born in Manali, India. She attended the Central School for Tibetans, Bylakuppe, South India, and later graduated from the Tibetan Medical and Astrological Institute in Dharamsala, India. She worked in the Tibetan Medical and Astrological Institute in New Delhi for three years, and then as Chief Medical Officer in Bhubneshwar, Orissa, India. She studied under Kunga Gurmey Nyarongsher, as well as Tenzin Choedak, senior personal physician to His Holiness the Dalai Lama. She lives in London, where she practices Tibetan medicine, and is the first Tibetan doctor resident in Great Britain.

Dr. Kseniya M. Gerasimova graduated from both the Leningrad Institute of Culture and Leningrad University. She also earned Ph.D.s from Leningrad University and from the Institute of Ethnography of the Russian Academy of Sciences in Moscow. A prominent Russian scholar in the field of Buddhist studies, she works in the Institute of Social Sciences of the Siberian Branch of the Russian Academy of Sciences in Moscow, and in the Institute of Social Sciences of the Siberian Branch of the Russian Academy of Sciences in Ulan-Ude. She has written seven monographs and more than a hundred twenty articles dealing with aspects of Buryat, Mongolian, and Tibetan culture.

H. H. The Dalai Lama, Tenzin Byatso, the 14th Dalai Lama and Nobel Peace Laureate, is considered the political and spiritual leader of the Tibetan people. Since his exile from Tibet in 1959, His Holiness has established a Tibetan Government in Dharamsala, India, where his efforts are concentrated on the preservation of the many facets of Tibetan culture. He is recognized and admired as a world leader for his commitment to non-violence, and has a large following worldwide.

Fernand Mayer, M.D., a physician and scholar, also serves as director for the research team for the environments, societies, and cultures of the Himalayas at the Centre National de la Recherche Scientifique. He teaches Tibetan history and culture at the Institut National des Langues et Civilizations Orientales, as well as traditional medicines of Asia at the Sorbonne, where he holds a Chair. Mayer has been conducting field work in Nepal, Bhutan, and Tibet since 1974, and has published extensively on Asian medicines, Tibetan art, architecture, and culture.